# RACE AGAINST THE ODDS

# ODDS

*The Tragic Success Story of Miss England II*

Kevin Desmond

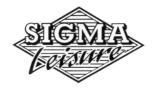

**Published by** Sigma Leisure – an imprint of Sigma Press, 5 Alton Road, Wilmslow, Cheshire SK9 5DY, England.

**British Library Cataloguing in Publication Data**
A CIP record for this book is available from the British Library.

**ISBN:** 1-85058-806-6


**Typesetting and Design by:** Sigma Press, Wilmslow, Cheshire.

**Printed by:** Interprint Ltd, Malta


**Cover Design:** Sigma Press, based on the painting of *Miss England II* by Arthur Benjamins

# Preface

During 30 years of research into world powerboating history, two speedboats have continued to intrigue me. Without doubt, Donald Campbell's legendary *Bluebird K7* jet-engined hydroplane remains a focal point for those who may know little of this minority sport. But the very first article about powerboat history which I managed to get accepted for publication was about *Miss England II*. This was in April 1974, the first of a series called 'Yesterday' and I was an enthusiastic 24-year-old.

But why *Miss England II*? In terms of achievement, this powerboat only broke the World Speed Record three times, lifting the speed by just 15 mph – as opposed to *Bluebird K7*'s total increase of 100 mph, and she failed to bring back the coveted bronze trophy for which she had been most expensively built.

Nevertheless, the quest to find out more and more about her was, for me, to become almost an obsession, but a fascinating one. Her fascination comes from the fact that she was the symbol of an extraordinary epoch. When this elegant projectile, representing the cream of the British Empire's technology and driven by one of her most admired Speed Kings came to grief, it was regarded as a national disaster. When she went to Argentina to lift the record, the Argentine Navy turned out to dredge the local River Parana. When she went to Italy, she was extravagantly fêted by Mussolini's arch rival, a poet called d'Annunzio. When she overturned again during a race watched by 600,000 spectators in Detroit, during the Prohibition era, a public accusation of trickery was made which has since gone down as one of the major controversies of boating history. No one boat indirectly promoted the presentation of two separate trophies or encouraged the Spiritualist movement. No one speedboat has ever inspired a full-length book.

My background reading was based on the fine biography of Sir Henry Segrave by the late Cyril Posthumus, who always encouraged and advised me in my quest. And, although my research concerned events which had taken place forty years before, back in the early 1970s a number of players and eye-witnesses were still living, although some were more ready to help than others.

Up at Windermere, I met George Pattinson, founder of the Windermere Steamboat Museum. As a teenager, George was an eyewitness to this tragically successful record-attempt. Indeed his father and uncle were Course Marshals. Like so many other eyewitnesses, George told me of the eerie silence in the seconds following the crash – eerie because there must have been almost one hundred spectator craft on Windermere.

Michael J. Willcocks had supervised construction of the hydroplane at Cowes and was her riding mechanic before – and very courageously after – the fatal accident on Windermere. He was still living in Clevedon, Somerset, next to the family engineering business, whence he applied for the task of riding mechanic in the cockpit of what was to be Britain's most powerful and innovative speedboat to-date. During the mid-1970s, I went down several times to interview "Wilkie" on audio tape and received a succession of fascinating letters, punched out on an old typewriter or in spindly barely readable handwriting, but giving detail after detail about what had been the greatest adventure of his life. Wilkie still had framed photos of speedboat aces Gar Wood and Betty Carstairs on the walls of his office, as well as the wickerwork seat Sir Henry Segrave had sat in on that fateful Friday 13th June 1930 when *Miss England II* hit a submerged log at an unprecedented 120mph with fatal consequences. Willcocks was the sole survivor. Appreciating my enthusiasm, Michael kindly gave me some unique and unpublished photographs. You'll find them in this book.

While on the subject of rare photos, keen to find anything possible about motorboat racing history, I placed an advertisement in a national daily newspaper. One response offered to sell me a photo of *Miss England II* on Thursday, June 12th 1930, autographed by her entire team. The following day, two crew were dead and the boat was on the lake bed. Although I bought this for the then princely sum of £20, subsequent penury, albeit temporary, forced me to re-sell it, for £30, to the Windermere Motor Boat Racing Club. (Twenty-five years later, the Club has kindly given me permission to use it in these pages.)

I also received this touching offer from Grange-over-Sands:

Dear Mr Desmond,

I have read your letter in "The Westmorland Gazette" regarding motor-boat speed records. I have a large number of press cuttings of the late Sir Henry Segrave, including press photographs, and graphic accounts of the speed attempt which ended in tragedy….These cuttings are stuck in a scrap-book and although perhaps somewhat childish, they are genuine, authentic and collected by me from local newspapers 1929/1930…. As a young girl, Sir Henry was a great hero of mine. I would like to think they could be of help to someone.

Yours sincerely,

Miss V Foster Ring

As for the other riding mechanic, Victor Halliwell, who lost his life in the record attempt, several years ago his son visited The Motorboat Museum at Basildon and loaned us some very fine photographs in memory of a father whom he had lost when only a child, but whose loss had forever after made him an over-cautious person.

Dick Garner, who retired to Nantwich, Cheshire, invited me into his home and told me about his tasks as riding mechanic in *Miss England II* when replacement driver Kaye Don won the first heat of the Harmsworth Trophy race in September 1931 – but was then "tricked" over the starting line and *Miss England II* crashed again, in one of the most controversial powerboat heats in the sport's history. Garner well remembered Detroit during Prohibition. He also gave me some splendid contemporary photos which he had brought home from the USA. Sadly, Dick died of a heart attack soon after our meeting.

Although Kaye Don was still alive, he wrote me a terse reply that, as it was his intention to write his own memoirs, he was unable to help me. He never did write those memoirs.

As for the boat's designer, Fred Cooper, to this day I regret not having persisted in trying to see him, even though he sent me this modest letter from Brading, Isle of Wight:

May 6th, 1970.

Dear Sir,

Thank you for your letter of the 2nd inst; and it will not be necessary for me to answer your questionnaire, which I return herewith, as I refer you to works by my great friend Uffa Fox.

Yours faithfully

Fred Cooper

When I later decided to try again, Cooper's widow told me that it had taken her a whole week to get rid of his papers on the garden bonfire! On the other hand, Mike Evans of the Rolls-Royce Heritage Trust in Derby found me a fine batch of photos of the *Miss England II* adventure.

As time passed, I found myself in the same places where the sweet drone of the black-bottomed bombshell's twin Rolls-Royce R aero-units had once thrilled huge crowds of spectators. In June 1980, I was out in Detroit. By this time, the 1931 Harmsworth defender, *Miss America IX* had been purchased and restored by Harold Mistele. One afternoon, during the weekend races for the APBA Gold Cup, Harold's son Chuck "took me for a spin" in *Miss America IX* around the Detroit River course, watched by 400,000 spectators. Thus, I experienced almost the same course as *Miss England II* had taken half a century before.

In May 1995, I was asked out to Lake Garda as a judge for a Classic Motorboat Rally. Not only did organiser Angelo Vassena give me a ride across that Italian lake where *Miss England II* had once lifted the World Water Speed Record, but his brother also took me to Gabriele d'Annunzio's lakeside palazzo "Vittoriale". Here, in the Room of the Leper, I saw Segrave's twisted steering wheel on display, surrounded by statuettes of Buddhas, Hindu gods and Holy Icons – a strange contrast.

My researches were never quite complete. Returning to Windermere in the 1990s, I called in at the local police station where the officer on duty managed to find the original hand-written police report of the events of 13th June 1930.

One of the great mysteries was the ultimate fate of *Miss England II*'s hull, after her second spectacular crash in Detroit. Some told me that she was languishing in a barn in Yorkshire, while others that she was in Norfolk. Ultimately, it was the local historian of Hounslow District Council who unearthed a tell-tale paragraph published in the local newspaper during the Blitz – its facsimile is published in this book.

About a year ago, I left my home near Bordeaux to join the celebrations of the 15th anniversary of The Motorboat Museum. Imagine my surprise when during the reception in the marquee, I was introduced to Roy Fisher, the son of Tommy Fisher, one of the Rolls-Royce mechanics on the *Miss England II* projects. Soon after, copies of three of Tommy's snapshots further enriched my collection.

I suppose my hobby could have remained a private obsession. But then my friend, Steve Holter, whose finely researched Campbell book "Leap into Legend" had just been published, suggested I offer my manuscript to his publisher Graham Beech of Sigma Press in Cheshire.

Apart from writing magazine articles about *Miss England II*, it gave me great pleasure to help others in their personal hobbies. Arthur Benjamins borrowed several photographs to create the splendid painting you'll find on the front cover of the book. Equally Fred Harris of Replicast Models benefited from those same photographs to create, firstly, a popular construction kit of *Miss England II* and later, three, 1-metre models. You can see one of these with "yours truly" on the back of the book.

Just before these pages went to press, I was interviewed by Flashback Television of London for a Channel 4 documentary called "Speed Kings". Imagine my fascination seeing long-forgotten newsreel footage of my favourite speedboat and actually hearing her R-types roaring into action once again!

In the sixty years which have followed the *Miss England II* adventure, powerboat racing and record-breaking have accelerated in leaps and bounds. The World Water Speed Record now stands at over 300 mph, three times the record speeds of Sir Henry Segrave, Kaye Don and Gar Wood. In the USA, aero-engined powerboats, competing for the APBA Gold Cup, accelerate along the straights at 200 mph and corner at 190. Race propellers regularly turn at speeds around 12,000rpm without breakage.

That said, rather like Telstar was the world's first communications satellite, *Miss England II*, the first speedboat to cross the 100 mph barrier, will always occupy a unique place in the history of sport. But the saga of *Miss England II* is not only about a speedboat. It is a profoundly human saga. I do hope you enjoy reading my researches ... so far, of course!

*Kevin Desmond*

*Bordeaux, France*

## Dedication

To my family,
for all their encouragement
over the years.

# Contents

# 1

## The Defender

This book tells the story of a very British speedboat called *Miss England II*. To understand the reason for her creation, we must first look into the life of the American speedboat ace, whose *Miss America* powerboats she was built to beat. His name was Gar Wood.

It was in the 1870s when Walter Willis Wood, who had run away from home at 14 to become a drummer boy in the Civil War, settled down with his wife Elizabeth to raise a family. Their son, Garfield Arthur was named after the President and Vice-President who were inaugurated in the year of his birth (December 4th, 1880), and he was one of 13 brothers and sisters. Little Gar's first job was to tend the neighbour's cows in Mapleton, Indiana, where he was born and where his father ran a grocery store. He offered to tend them for 2 cents per cow per month; he got the job and 20 cows to herd. His father, meanwhile, pushed a variety of enterprises – store-keeping, farming, railroad work, woodcutting during the winters, and later, in Minnesota, operating a ferryboat.

On Lake Osakis, Minnesota, the boy was crewing on his father's excursion and ferryboat *Manitoba*. Rivalry was intense between Walt Wood and the captain of another ferry, *Belle of Osakis*, one Wes Mann, whose supreme ambition was to demonstrate that the *Belle* was the fastest boat on the lake. Both were wood-burning steam paddleboats, and one day they met in a race that was to have meaning beyond the little world of the upper Midwest's lakes. Walt Wood was startled to find that he was short of fuel. Wes Mann, pushing his boat under a plume of smoke, churned into the lead, giving a Minneapolis cheer as he went by. Walt Wood shouted back and then asked little Gar to give him a hand in breaking up the boat's furniture. Father and son dismembered chairs and tables in wild haste as their boat got up a furious finish and won.

"I still feel a thrill of winning that race," said Gar Wood, decades later. "The engines driving those paddlewheels fascinated me. I resolved right then that someday I was going to build and race boats of my own."

Before he reached his teens, Gar knew a good deal about boats and engines. He made a series of toy boats with clockwork motors, and one of the hottest rows he ever had with his father followed his dissection of the family alarm clock to make a tiny powerplant. He retrieved the situation by selling the toy boat for more than the clock cost. By this time the family had moved to Duluth, on the shores of the great Lake Superior and, at the age of 13, Gar Wood was a professional skipper, running the first gasoline-engined launch ever seen in Duluth.

"My first speed craft was a 16ft boat with a three-horsepower engine," he later told a journalist. "With it I succeeded in getting 8mph running up and down the harbour at Duluth near my home, merely by squirting raw gasoline into the bell of the motor with an oil can. Soon after, I built a boat for Dick Schell of Duluth. He had a 10-hp engine, and its 15mph made it the fastest motorboat in this country, perhaps the fastest in the world. We beat all the other boats on Lake Minnetonka at Minneapolis."

Fred W. Dingle, a St Paul boatbuilder, put together a boat in those years called *Fritz* for a man at Duluth. When Gar saw *Fritz*'s superior performance, he went to St Paul to talk to the man who could build such a boat. Soon after, Gar Wood moved to St Paul, taking with him his new bride, Murlen. In St Paul, this mechanical hobbyist from the lake country started a kind of portable repair shop, going around town fixing broken automobiles, and often dropping in at Dingle's boatyard to talk speedboats. "Gar Wood was a likeable boy, and although many of his ideas were crazy, he managed to think things out and get rid of the freak plans such as a narrow boat with a gyroscope as stabilizer," said a man who knew him on the waterfront in those early, speedboat-mad years of the twentieth century.

In 1911, financed by W.P. Cleveland, Gar built a boat called *Leading Lady* in a machine shop he had opened. The engine was bulky and the hull was crude-looking, but *Leading Lady* had the speed. He took her to the Mississippi Valley Powerboat Association's regatta at Duluth, and succeeded in covering ten miles at a 30mph average – excellent performance for a small boat in that year when the fastest boat in the world, a 50ft hydroplane with 800 horsepower was just breaking the 50mph barrier. The following year, having modified an already successful hull, Messrs. Wood and Cleveland went to a succession of races in the Midwest and cleaned up. Gar had the skills to do great things; now all he needed was money.

One day in 1912, in St Paul, Wood saw a truck driver in St Peter Street unloading two tons of coal with a hand-operated lift and cursing the heavy dirty work. Surely, he thought, there must be an easier way to unload coal. "Mrs Wood and I had just $200 between us at the time," he recalled. "'I've got a new idea,' I told her one day, 'a mechanical device for dumping trucks. Shall I put the money in it?' She was a good sport and said to go ahead – that $200 would not make or break us." Wood used half of this nest egg. He built the world's first hydraulic hoist in a backyard garage, using a cylinder he bought for 50 cents in a scrapyard, making the gear system himself, and borrowing the truck from the coal man he had seen on the street.

"The owner of the truck and a group of other men, who had been attending a party, heard of our experiment one night, and hurried to the garage. We were all ready for the final job. Most of them were top-hatted and in formal dress; but they climbed into the truck body and we started the hoist. It shot up too fast and rolled a dozen well-dressed gentlemen unceremoniously onto the floor. They took it good-naturedly enough, and there was immediate demand for the device. We patented it and started a business, the Wood Hydraulic Hoist and Body Company. It grew so quickly that I soon brought my brothers into the business to help out. It was the year father died."

The business was to grow so nicely that Gar Wood was always assured of an income to support his insatiable enthusiasm for newer and faster speedboats. Indeed, in 1912, he was already flush enough to buy an engine from his former client, Cleveland, and install it in his own hull, which he named the *Little Leading Lady*.

In those early racing days, Mrs Wood brought a toy teddy bear for 15 cents in St Paul. Gar stole it from her as his mascot to carry aboard *Little Leading Lady*, and the boat won all the races for which she was eligible in the Mississippi Valley Powerboat Association's big regatta at Keokuk. Murlen brought another teddy bear. Gar stole that one, too. Teddy and Bruin became riding mates and much more. For the next two decades, without Teddy and Bruin aboard, Gar Wood would not race. All the dollars in the world could not buy them. Murlen Wood was soon making tiny cork lifejackets, bathing caps, ear mufflers and rubber-soled shoes for these treasured racing companions. As speeds on the water escalated, Gar's trust in the magic of Teddy and Bruin became even stronger – obsessive almost. "They are the captains of my fate," he once remarked.

In 1914, Gar Wood, Murlen Wood, family and business moved to Detroit. That summer, once again, he won all the Mississippi Valley races at Peoria. Enter Christopher Columbus Smith, the renowned backwoods boatbuilder from Algonac, 40 miles north of Detroit. He had been creating raceboats since 1911, first for John 'Baldy' Ryan, a St Louis and Cincinnati sportsman, then for J. Stuart Blackton, silent movie pioneer, then for the Miss Detroit Powerboat Association, whose 250hp Sterling-engined *Miss Detroit I* swept all three heats of the 1915 contest for the Gold Cup, America's most coveted powerboat trophy. But because that association was unable to raise the money to pay Chris Smith for a new *Miss Detroit* for 1916, *Miss Minneapolis*, another boat Chris Smith had built for a group of Minneapolis sportsmen, walked home with American powerboating's most prestigious trophy. The impecunious group in Detroit was faced with the problem of selling *Miss Detroit I*, now an outclassed white elephant, to the highest bidder.

The bidder was Gar Wood. He not only bought the boat, he bought into Chris Smith's boatbuilding yard and commissioned *Miss Detroit III*, the hydroplane he drove with Jay Smith to win the Gold Cup in 1917. Gar Wood was now in the big leagues of powerboat racing, and he began to give it all he had. He became the first U.S. racingman to put an aircraft engine, a 12-cylinder Curtiss V-type, into a boat, *Miss Detroit III*. The experts considered him mad.

The 1918 Gold Cup race was something of a family affair. Gar Wood and Jay Smith in *Miss Detroit III*, George Wood and

Bernard Smith in *Miss Detroit II*, Winfield and Louis Wood in *Miss Minneapolis*. Their father, Captain Walt, would have been proud. Despite being burnt by the flames shooting from the exhaust stacks of the *III*, Gar Wood defended the Gold Cup and kept it Detroit. He also won the prestigious Thousand Islands Trophy that season. On the strength of these victories, and the weakness of prices for surplus engines after World War I, the Detroit Marine Aero Engine Company was formed, purchasing a quantity of Fiat, Benz, Mercedes, Liberty and Beardmore aircraft engines. Before long, almost every high-speed power-boat in the U.S. had one or more of these engines. As Gar Wood's nephew, Walter W. Wood of Grosse Pointe, recalled: "I remember Detroit Marine Aero Engine Company as a warehouse with crated engines stacked three or four high. Most were Libertys – built by Packard, Ford, Marmon Herrington, and others. I remember my father remarking that Liberty engines could be had for less than the price of the cheapest hoist and body."

Another successful defence of the Gold Cup was made in 1919 by *Miss Detroit III*. Ever ambitious, Wood now sought the most coveted prize in powerboat racing – the British International (Harmsworth) Trophy. Its rules specified that every aspect of a competing boat must be national – pilot, mechanic, engines, and hull. Wood had been building his boats of British Honduras mahogany, and now he changed over to Philippine mahogany. From using German Bosch magnetos, he switched to American electrical equipment. This time his Liberty 12-cylinder engines, developed from an early Mercedes racing-car powerplant, used in the First World War to push de Havilland DH-4 aeroplanes, and modified after the war to deliver 500 and more horsepower, were to be used – two per boat. Gar Wood fielded the 38ft *Miss Detroit V* for rough-water racing and the 26ft *Miss America I* for smooth water. Both hulls were designed and built by Chris Smith. Gar took both to Southampton Waters in England and, in August 1920, averaging 61mph, he won the two heats necessary to take the bronze Harmsworth Trophy back to Detroit. On his return, he went out in *Miss America I* and successfully defended the Gold Cup, averaging 70mph for three heats – a Gold Cup record that would not be eclipsed until after World War II.

Gar now took another step with his boats and put no fewer than four of his Grant-Liberty engines, totalling 2000 horsepower, in the new *Miss America II*. Experts considered her a vehicle destined to break up, blow up or take to the air like one of the new seaplanes. But he had little trouble with the new machine – something that would characterise most of his racing and record-setting – and no trouble defending the 1921 Harmsworth Trophy from Britain's Col. A.W. Tate, driving the 1800hp *Maple Leaf VII*, which had been dropped accidentally from a crane and whose engines were out of alignment. As a sporting gesture between heats, Gar's mechanics helped the English team in their efforts to repair the boat – in vain. Soon after, *Miss America II* was clocked at 80.57mph in the Mile Championships of North America. This was the beginning of Wood's dream to become the first man to travel 100mph on the water.

Also in 1921, the Detroit Yacht Club decided to build the finest plant in the world on Belle Isle. They elected Gar Wood as Commodore, an honour he was to keep for the next half century. Businesswise, the Commodore continued to prosper with his hydraulic hoist business: three factories in Detroit, one in Windsor, Ontario, and even an assembly plant in Paris. He also began to build a line of gentlemen's speedboats, offshoots of his racing hulls that were the Buicks or stock runabouts in the Roaring Twenties – Chris-Craft boats being the Chevrolets and Pontiacs, and John Hacker's boats, the Packards.

During the winter of 1921/22, the American Power Boat Association (APBA) decided that in future, entries for the Gold Cup should be limited to displacement boats of more than 25ft and with engines of not more than 625 cubic-inch displacement. The intention was to encourage a high standard of gentlemen's runabouts, raceboats that would be useful for amusements other than competition. Extreme aero-engined hydroplanes such as *Miss America* were being discouraged.

This annoyed Gar Wood. He felt that the APBA was trying to break his stranglehold on the Gold Cup. Which it did, because the 1922 contest was won by Col. Jesse G. Vincent's *Packard Chris-Craft*, built by Chris Smith, who had also built *Baby Gar Jr*, the boat Gar Wood drove to third place. It was the first race Gar Wood had lost in years. That Chris Smith should betray him by building a quicker boat for Colonel Vincent was hard to believe. It was the beginning of an estrangement. Although he raced *Curtis Baby Gar* in 1923, and *Baby America* in 1924, Wood was never able to regain his hold on the APBA Gold Cup.

In 1923, to counter the APBA restrictions, Messrs. Wood and Chapman cleverly formed the Yachtsman's Association of America (YAA) and organised a long-distance International Sweepstakes Race for $25,000 at Detroit. For the first contest, Chris Smith built *Packard Chris-Craft II*, *Packard Chris-Craft III* and *Miss Packard* for Jesse Vincent. Gar's new boatbuilder, Joseph Napoleon 'Nap' Lisée, a 52-year-old New Yorker and former employee of Chris Smith, built two new boats called *Teddy* and *Bruin*. The little town of Algonac was split down the middle in its support – either for Chris Smith or Gar Wood. The race covered 50 three-mile laps. Vincent's *Packard Chris-Craft II* developed mechanical glitches after leading for the first 32 laps. *Teddy*, driven by brother George Wood, forged into the lead and finished in that position. There was, however, a snag. *Teddy* was racing without her engine-hatch covers from lap 34 and recovered them on lap 45. Vincent protested, backed up by Chris Smith. Tempers were lost. Hasty words were spoken. Gar Wood stood up in the dining room of the Detroit Yacht Club that evening and, in his capacity as an official of the YAA, vehemently overruled Colonel Vincent's protest. The following day the YAA race committee handed in a blanket resignation. The whole thing was a fiasco.

During the next two decades, the two Algonac companies, fierce in rivalry, were to produce an ever-increasing range of fast runabouts, commuter cruisers and sportsboats. Had Chris Smith and Gar Wood not split in 1923, it is interesting to speculate whether there might not have been one company instead of two, playing a key role in the mahogany runabout market of the 1920s.

In 1924, Gar got his own back on the APBA. The Fisher-Allison Trophy had been offered for gentlemen's runabouts. Wood's previous entries had been ruled out of two Fisher-Allison contests because the rules prohibited the use of aircraft engines. His opposition finally backed down a bit and decreed that any boat with engine specs up to 1050 cubic inches could enter. But the opposition joked that "no gentleman would ever drive in one of those boats." Wood and his riding mechanic, Orlin Johnson, showed up at Buffalo for the Fisher-Allison test in white tie and tails, their top hats secured by strings under their chins. Even the two teddy-bear mascots were in evening dress. They won, going away in *Baby Gar IV* and sliding up to the judge's stand as immaculate as when they started. "You see, this really is a gentleman's boat," quipped Wood as he accepted the trophy.

The next year, in May, 1925, Richard F. Hoyt having chosen his weather and tide conditions, raced his boat *Teaser* against the New York Central's celebrated 'Twentieth Century Ltd' express train from Albany to New York. He covered the 138 miles in 160 minutes. A week later, Commodore Wood and brother George climbed into *Baby Gar IV* and *Baby Gar V* in an attempt to better that record. Gar actually challenged Hoyt to race down the Hudson, betting $25,000 to beat him. Hoyt refused, saying that his boat was built for commuting, not racing. Although *Baby Gar IV* beat the train by 38 minutes and averaged 46.5mph over the mileage, burning only 110 gallons of gas, she was 18 minutes slower than *Teaser*'s time. Big crowds watched the run all the way down the river.

During the next decade, Gar was to have two obsessive speedboat-racing priorities: to defend his hold on the Harmsworth Trophy from increasingly powerful opposition, and to retain the title of World Water Speed Record holder. The Harmsworth contest was to grow into one of the major events of the North American sporting calendar. It is incredible to reflect how half a million people converged annually on Detroit in the twenties and early thirties to watch, in the far distance, never more than four of the world's fastest boats racing round a course for less than half an hour. But so it was.

In 1925, Henri Esdres challenged with *Excelsior-France*. Gar Wood had just written off *Miss America II*, which he crashed into a tree at the side of Florida's Indian River at more than 50mph. He now built his '*III*' and '*IV*', modifying five new Liberty engines at a cost of $25,000. In an 80mph trial on Lake Geneva, *Excelsior-France* caught fire, and her two 16-cylinder Breguet engines sank to the bottom. The Harmsworth contest was cancelled and Gar Wood was left with two new boats he might never use.

In 1926, Esdres built *Excelsior-France II* and challenged again. Having learned that the new French boat was en route for the States, Wood built *Miss America V. Excelsior-France II*, driven by T.A. Clarke, and despite sporting help from Wood's mechanics, proved a hopeless and unreliable machine. She broke down in the race while Gar in his *V* beat his brothers George and Phil in the *III* and the *IV* in a family race. It was the following year that Commodore Gar Wood, aged 47, the fastest man in the world on the water, was introduced to the English Major Henry Segrave, 31 years old and the fastest man in the world on land. Segrave had just driven his Sunbeam SLUG down Daytona Beach at a record speed of 203mph.

The two record holders were both talking about speedboats. The US Commodore had just taken the British Major out for a spin in his *Miss America V*. They discussed the Harmsworth Trophy and the need for a real challenger. Segrave saw no reason why, with the necessary sponsorship, an all-British speedboat could not be put together with, for example, *Miss England* painted on her bows.

Before these two men parted, Wood bought a Sunbeam car from Segrave and the Englishman took an outboard engine back to Great Britain. To better understand why Gar Wood may well have met his match in Henry Segrave, we will now look at the equally adventuresome life of this potential Harmsworth challenger.

# 2

## The Challenger

Henry O'Neal de Hane Segrave was born in Baltimore, USA, on 22 December 1896 and was of Irish descent. In 1905, when he was only nine years old, he attempted to drive an automobile for the first time. He was scarcely able to reach the foot pedals. His parents did not realise that he was attempting to drive – even though his father was an amateur engineer with an early interest in cars and even though it was his father's car. During this initiation ceremony, Wilson, the Segrave's chauffeur – and young Henry's secret instructor – took fright at the speed his young pupil was doing. He promptly turned off the de Dietrich engine.

Henry was only ten years old when he had his first experience in driving his father's fast American motor launch around the local lake. This time his father was passenger, but the young man still cruised at a considerable speed. At the same time, the boy was building himself an increasingly complex indoor model railway – possibly the biggest in Southern Ireland, where his family was living at the time.

At the outbreak of war, Segrave was at Eton Public School and thence entered Sandhurst. He was gazetted to the post of lieutenant in the First Battalion the Royal Warwickshire Regiment and, in December 1914, rushed out to the Western Front. On May 17th 1915 he was shot in a hand-to-hand encounter in what was mistakenly thought to be an abandoned German trench. Segrave was rescued by men of his own battalion and taken back behind the lines. For days he was near death. He was sent back to England, convalesced and before long was learning to fly in a Maurice Farman biplane at the Central Flying School, Upavon. His Royal Aero Club Certificate number 2090 was dated November 19th 1915. In 1916 he married Miss Doris

Stocker, who was one of the most charming and competent young musical comedy actresses of the time.

Segrave was seconded to the Royal Flying Corps in January 1916 and served in England with No. 19 and No. 32 Squadrons before being posted overseas to No. 29 Squadron in April 1916. He was appointed Flight Commander in May 1916 and posted to HQ British Expeditionary Force. Before the end of 1916 he had been wounded three times and, in his last crash, he had brought down four enemy aircraft before his own ship, an FE8 Scout, was riddled with enemy bullets. His broken body was found at dusk, slumped in a battered cockpit in a tree; one of his legs was so badly damaged that it left him with a permanent injury. But he lived and was soon posted, in January 1917, to the War Office with the temporary rank of Captain.

In May 1918 he was appointed to the Department of the Chief of the Air Staff, Air Ministry, where he was Technical Secretary to Lord Rothermere who was then Air Minister. Later that year, Major Segrave was attached to the British Aviation Mission, Washington, which went to America to help the development of Military Aviation in the United States. In this he was very successful, partly because of his American birth and partly by virtue of his own personality. Whilst out in the States, Segrave caught the motor-racing bug when he took part in a race at Sheepshead Bay Track on Long Island and lapped an Apperson at 82mph. When his Mission wanted to get home, shipping was scarce. Women were not allowed to travel on the Atlantic lines, the import of motor-cars was forbidden, and dogs from foreign countries were not admitted to Great Britain under any conditions. But young Henry Segrave, then 23 years of age, arrived smiling from the States with his wife, a large American automobile, and a pure-bred British bulldog. When he was asked how he had managed this, Segrave just laughed in that way he had when he was treating anything difficult as a rather good joke, and said, "It was quite easy when you knew how ..."

After the Armistice, Segrave left the Royal Air Force and turned his attention to motor-racing. He tried to get a place on the STD (Sunbeam-Talbot-Darracq) team but due to his lack of experience he was politely turned down. His first drive in 1920 was in a pre-war Opel single-seater at the Brooklands Track. In this first race, a wheel flew off at more than 100mph. Exhibiting tremendous coolness and skill, Segrave held the car steady and came safely to a halt. Just 45 minutes later, using the same car, he entered his second race and registered his first victory. Following two more wins, three seconds and three thirds that season, Segrave managed to obtain a place on the STD team – albeit driving the *fourth* car.

In the six years that followed, driving Sunbeam and Talbot cars, he had been positioned in forty-four of the races which he had entered, coming first in thirty-one of them. Among eight major victories were the British, Spanish and French Grand Prix. His victory in the 1923 French Grand Prix, then regarded as the world's top motor-race, marked the first time in history that a Grand Prix had been won by a British driver.

During 1926, Segrave decided to attack the World Land Speed Record. The Sunbeam Motor Company had built a V12 4-litre car, designed especially for the task by Louis Coätelen. Segrave 'enjoyed' some bumpy rides along Southport Sands before he broke the existing record at a speed of 152.33mph.

In 1927, he decided to retire from motor-racing and set his sights on becoming the first man to travel at over 200mph on land. Sunbeams built a car powered by two 400hp Matabele aero-engines. Segrave took this to Daytona Beach, Florida. Despite nearly swerving into the Atlantic breakers, he managed to clock 203.79mph.

It was during this time that Gar Wood gave Segrave that exhilarating ride in *Miss America V* and suggested that he might like to make an attempt to wrest the Harmsworth Trophy from him.

Returning to England with the American outboard engine as part of his baggage, Segrave publicly announced his intention of taking up motorboat racing as a hobby. In May 1927 at the Hythe Regatta, he had won his first motor-boat race at 17.9 knots in his 8-horsepower outboard dinghy, *Meteorite*.

During the months that followed Segrave got in a great deal of experience and fun in regatta races, so that by 1928, he was ready to challenge America. For sponsorship of both the car and the boat, Segrave immediately turned to the one man capable of footing such a hefty bill: Sir Charles Wakefield of the Castrol Oil Company.

# 3

# The Patron

Charles Cheers Wakefield was born in Liverpool on December 12th 1859, the youngest son of an HM Customs officer. Educated at the Liverpool Institute, he entered the office of an oil broker and made several journeys around the world. In 1883, he married Sarah Frances Graham; they were to remain childless.

In 1891, he came to London and was associated with a great American corporation dealing in oil. In 1899, aged forty, he founded the firm of C.C. Wakefield and Co. The office then comprised three rooms on the top floor of 27 Cannon Street, London, and the total staff numbered nine. For the first six or seven years sales were confined mainly to railway oils. No records exist to show exactly when a lubricating oil was introduced for the comparatively new-fangled petrol engine, but it was sometime during 1906. For the next two years, Wakefield Motor Oil, as it was called, was sold on a limited scale, its largest user being the Vanguard Bus Company, who operated one of the earliest London passenger services.

In 1909, the recently knighted Sir Charles Wakefield decided to make a serious attempt to enter the motor and aero oil markets. At that time there were only some 48,000 cars and 35,000 motor-cycles on the road and flying was in its infancy, but Wakefield foresaw the vast possibilities that lay ahead. His first step was to provide Wakefield Motor Oil with a distinctive brand name – and so Wakefield Motor Oil's 'Castrol' brand (so-called because castor oil was an ingredient) was brought into being.

In October 1909, the first aero meeting in this country was held at Doncaster and every event was won on Castrol R. Sir Charles understood very well the value of publicity and, from the outset, he ensured that every Castrol success was brought to the attention of the public. The flights of the pioneer airmen, the winning of the Isle of Man senior T.T. races of 1911, 1912, 1913, and Hornsted's 128mph Land Speed Record were typical subjects of Castrol advertisements of the period. An aura of romance and glamour was built up around the name Castrol, and this was to be one of the company's greatest assets.

Wakefield made use of the boom in the automobile industry, dealing in lubricating oils and appliances. Combining this with a faculty for choosing the right technical experts and an appreciation of the value of publicity rapidly brought him great wealth. The sales of the new oil increased beyond all expectations and, by 1913, it was necessary to move to large offices at Wakefield House in Cheapside.

With the outbreak of war in 1914, Castrol was in demand by all the fighting services, but in particular by the Royal Flying Corps, as 'R' was one of the few oils suitable for the rotary-engined planes then in use. From these war years comes what must be the strangest testimonial ever received by an oil company. One of the British Handley Page bombers had the misfortune to land intact behind the German lines. It was inspected by the Kaiser and made a high level flight in his presence. According to an eye-witness, the Kaiser turned to his Chief of Staff, General Hoppner, and asked, "How is it that at such a height on such a cold day the lubricant does not freeze?" The General replied, "The British have discovered the secret which we have been seeking for months." The machine was fitted with Rolls-Royce engines and was using Castrol 'R'.

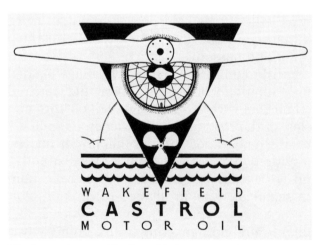

The famous logo used by Castrol Ltd in its annual "Achievement Books". *(Burmah-Castrol)*

14

Needless to say, this unique testimonial was put to effective use.

Between November 1915 and November 1916, Sir Charles Wakefield as Lord Mayor of London, threw himself wholeheartedly into the work of recruiting, daily addressing crowds from the balcony of the Mansion House or in the surrounding streets. Before he left office, he visited the London troops at the Western Front and the Grand Fleet at Scapa Flow. He placed his new residence at Hythe at the disposal of the Royal Army Service Corps. He was a great philanthropist where war charities were concerned, particularly hospitals and orphanages. At the close of his year of office, he received a baronetcy and two years later was made Companion of the British Empire.

During the war, racing and record breaking naturally came to an end and private motoring was much restricted. Mechanised farming, however, was just coming into vogue and, to meet the demand for a reliable tractor oil, Agricastrol, was put on the market in 1917. It, too, was a great success and by 1918 the Company was able to claim that 'Agricastrol' was being used by the majority of Fordson tractors then in operation. The end of the war in 1918 found the motor industry well established and, with the advent of mass production, there began a vast rise in the output of motor vehicles. In 1913 there had been 100,000 cars registered. This figure remained fairly constant throughout the war but, by 1922, car registrations had risen to 245,000 and those of motorcycles to 370,000. The market was expanding with a vengeance.

The 1920s were years of great achievement on land, sea and air, in which men vied with each other to travel further and faster than ever before with every form of mechanical transport. Sir Charles Wakefield, realising the technical importance of such exploits, became the driving force behind almost every British onslaught upon records and feats of endurance with aeroplanes, racing cars, motorcycles – and speedboats. He supported, with his money, the flights of Sir Alan Cobham to Australia and back, and his flight round Africa. He helped Miss Amy Johnson to make her famous flight to Australia. He provided Wakefield scholarships for the Royal Air Force Cadets at Cranwell. It was for such precedents that Segrave turned to

Wakefield as the logical sponsor for his attack on American speedboat supremacy.

At 71 years of age, Wakefield was a grim, dour, childless old man, with a somewhat nonconformist face, shrewd eyes, rat-trap mouth and fusty frock-coat. But he was a patriot and farsighted – and that is what counted.

# 4

# A Very British Speedboat

For a speedboat to beat Gar Wood, Lord Wakefield and Segrave now approached Hubert Scott-Paine, the far-sighted chief of the British Powerboat Company, and asked him to build a boat to accompany his new land-speed record car, the *Golden Arrow*, to Florida early in 1929. Like the *Golden Arrow*, the boat should be powered by the much proved Napier Lion aero-engine. This engine had powered the Supermarine S5 seaplane when it won the 1927 Schneider Trophy contest at Calshot.

Scott-Paine carefully explained his theory to Segrave who had to drive the boat. He was convinced that success lay in the design of smaller, single-engined boats and that trophies such as the Harmsworth would be brought back through the skilful driving of such boats rather than through the brute force of several marinised aero engines. He went on to demonstrate that breaking water speed records was unlike similar attempts either in the air or in motor cars.

The movement of water due to current and tide, the effects of wind, disturbances due to boats or even relatively distant ships, semi-submerged objects such as water-logged wood, all provided hazards even on a seemingly ideal day. Time after time, 'Scotty' told his audience, he had seen boats tearing along at 40 to 60mph, then hit some disturbance and jump high in the air. He went on to remind them that the newspapers were still covering the story of how the plucky Betty Carstairs and her mechanic had been thrown out of their *Estelle* hydroplane during the 1928 Harmsworth Trophy earlier that month. They had been lucky not to be killed. Even a flat calm could conceal a rise and fall due to a disturbance that perhaps originated many miles away.

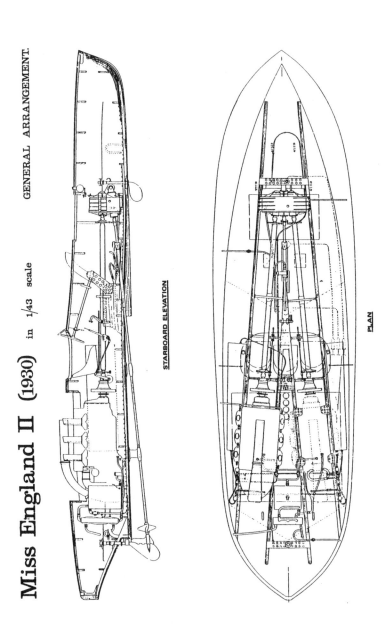

*Miss England II starboard elevation (Courtesy, Fred Harris and B.J. McLean)*

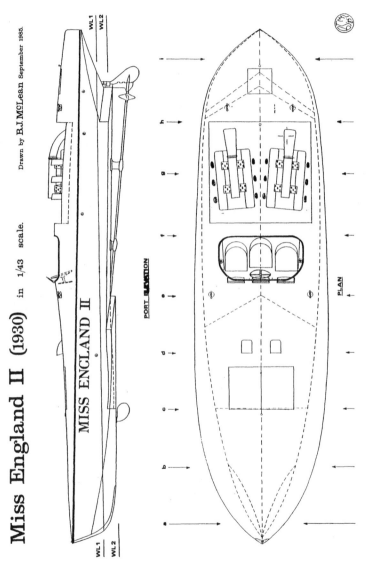

Miss England II (1930) in 1/43 scale.

Drawn by B.J. McLean September 1985.

MISS ENGLAND II

PORT ELEVATION

PLAN

WL 1
WL 2

*Miss England II port elevation (Courtesy, Fred Harris and B.J. McLean)*

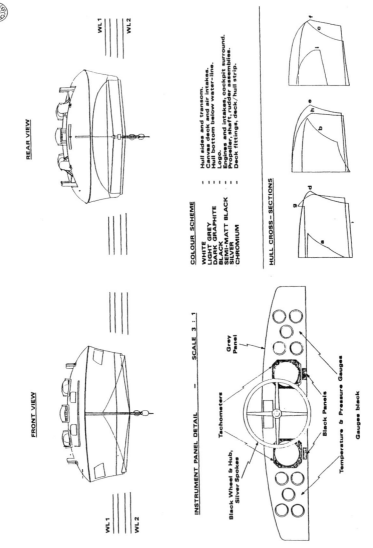

*Miss England II details (Courtesy, Fred Harris and B.J. McLean)*

During the 1927/28 season, Scott-Paine driving his 250hp Siddeley-Puma-engined *Panther P1* had won nine first prizes and two seconds in the eleven races for which he entered her. He therefore argued that Segrave's best chance of success lay in mastering the manoeuvrability of a small boat, and the skill in handling one propeller, designed for extremely high revs.

To realise the designs of such a challenger, Scott-Paine went to Hythe to talk with the promising naval architect, Fred Cooper. Two years younger than Segrave, Cooper's childhood ambition had been to become an aircraft designer. In this, the boy was dissuaded by his father, a monumental mason, who considered there was no financial future in 'flying machines'. Following studies at the Portman House Academy on the Isle of Wight, Cooper spent much of the war out in the Dardanelles as sub-lieutenant in the Royal Naval Voluntary Reserve.

On Armistice, after serving an apprenticeship with Thornycrofts at Basingstoke, Cooper learnt perfectionism in boatbuilding design and construction from Sidney E. Porter, chief draughtsman at S.E. Saunders Ltd. of East Cowes. One of Cooper's first raceboats was *Newg*, a 17ft single-step hydroplane powered by a 1.5 litre Sunbeam racing car engine – to be owner-driven by a brave 25-year-old millionairess called Marion Carstairs and her racing mechanic Joe Harris. In 1927, following two victorious seasons, Fred Cooper and Joe Harris campaigned *Newg* in the USA and won the first motorboat trophy Britain had brought back from the States in fifteen years.

Ably assisted by a recently recruited design assistant called Tommy Quelch, Cooper came up with a design for a 26ft single-step hydroplane with the engine mounted as far as possible against the transom, which thereby acted as a second riding step when the boat was at speed. The broad forward step acted as a balancer and carried relatively little weight so that there would be little tendency to submerge forward while the boat was at speed. The hull construction incorporated all of Scott-Paine's experience in motorboat racing and he naturally supervised the marine conversion of the Napier engine that was to drive a single propeller at a revolutionary 6,800 rpm. The unorthodox propeller was designed and made at Scott-Paine's British Power Boat Company at Hythe after 'Scotty' had conducted numerous experiments.

Many entirely novel features were designed, including a water-lubricated bearing for the tail shaft and a special water-cooling arrangement for the engine.

Scotty (Scott-Paine) drove his small band to work all hours while the boat was designed and built in the greatest secrecy at Hythe. The plans for the boat were completed on Tommy Quelch's drawing board in a remarkable three weeks and four days. The construction of the hull took only seven weeks and two days. It was a formidable achievement, but delays in the delivery of the engine meant that there was no time for trials before the boat had to be shipped to America. There was time, however, for a bit of publicity and Scotty took the diminutive racer to London for a special showing at Boots Ltd, Piccadilly. *Miss England* was then returned to Southampton and loaded on board the *RMS Majestic*, which was preparing to sail for New York on January 31st 1929.

That March, after establishing a new land speed record of 231.36mph in the *Golden Arrow*, Segrave started warming up *Miss England* to speeds of over 60mph, ready for their international motorboat duel with Gar Wood in *Miss America VII*. According to American journalist, James Lee Barrett in his pro-Gar Wood book 'Speed Boat Kings':

"After the land record, Wood went to Segrave and asked the Englishman to show him his boat and give him a demonstration of its performance. Upon looking at the boat when it was out of water Wood saw immediately that the propeller was too large and the bow rudder poorly designed. A test run of the boat proved both these factors to be true.

"The Committee at Miami Beach was anxious to have Segrave bring his boat to the annual Regatta and pit it against Wood's *Miss America VII*. In view of Wood's experienced criticism of his boat, Segrave did not know what to do, so Wood volunteered to send his crew of mechanics to Daytona Beach to put on a proper rudder and to furnish Segrave with suitable propellers. 'After considerable calculation of Segrave's horsepower and hull design, Wood ordered three propellers from the Hyde Company and gave them to Segrave. With a new rudder on his boat and with Wood's propellers, *Miss England I* was a very formidable, competitive boat. That's what Wood wanted. He wanted a good race ...'"

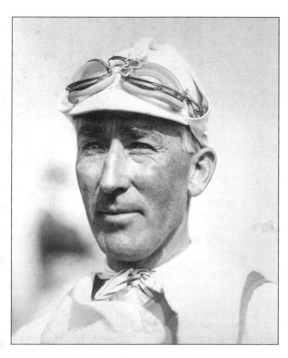

Left: Speed King Gar Wood *(Gar Wood collection)*

Below: Gar Wood with co-pilot Orlin Johnson on the twin-Packard engined *Miss America IX* at Indian Creek, their Florida testing ground during the late 1920s *(Author's Collection)*

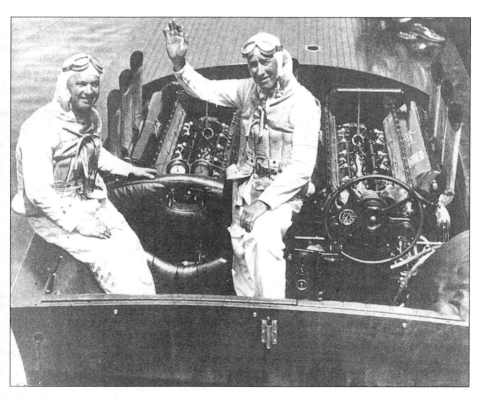

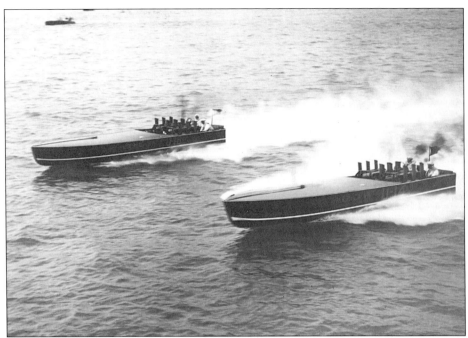

At speed, the Packard aero-engined *Miss America* boats were unbeatable *(Author's Collection)*

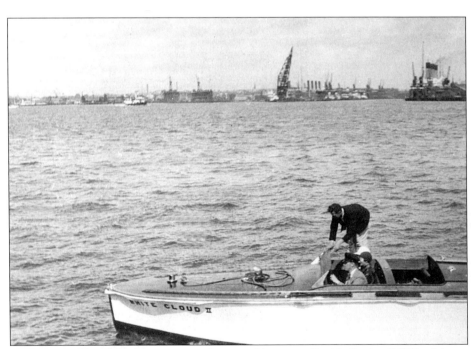

Segrave, with wife Doris as passenger, learns to drive a speedboat in Gordon Selfridge Jr.'s runabout *White Cloud II (Wynell-Mayow Lloyd Collection)*

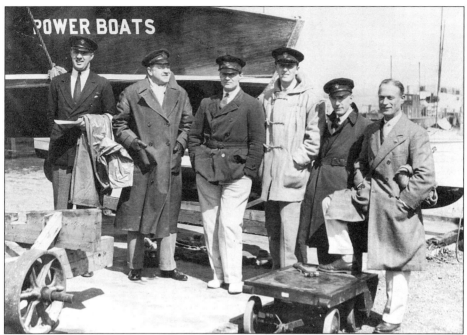

The team which created the first *Miss England*. Left to right: Lord Brecknock, Scott-Paine, Gordon Selfridge Jr., Segrave, Fred Cooper and Colonel Warwick Wright *(Quadrant Picture Library)*

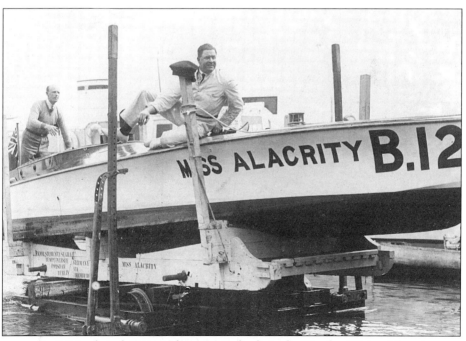

Scott-Paine for'ard, Segrave aft in *Miss England*'s tender *(Quadrant Picture Library)*

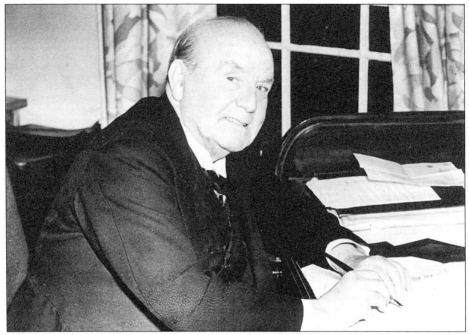

Lord Wakefield, founder head of Castrol Oil Company, and patron of record-breakers on land, air and water *(Burmah-Castrol)*

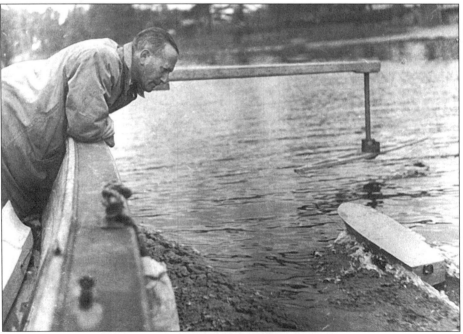

Fred Cooper testing a hull design *(Author's collection)*

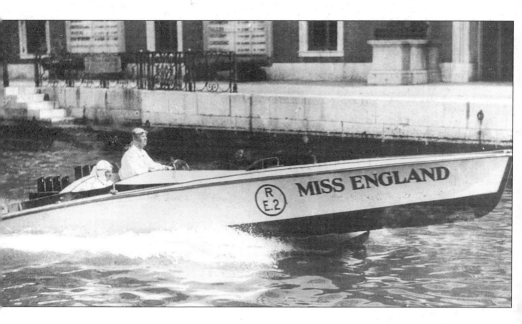

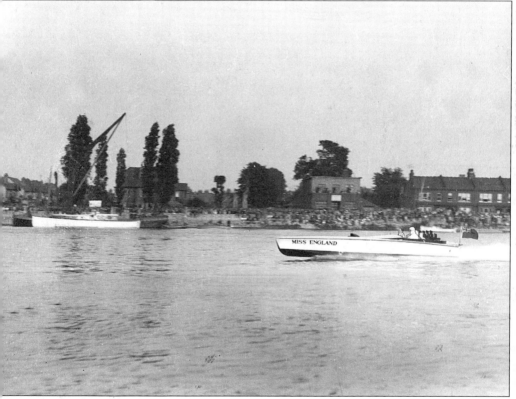

Top: *Miss England* at Venice, Segrave at the helm
Bottom: *Miss England* at speed on the Thames at Chelsea *(Quadrant Picture Library)*

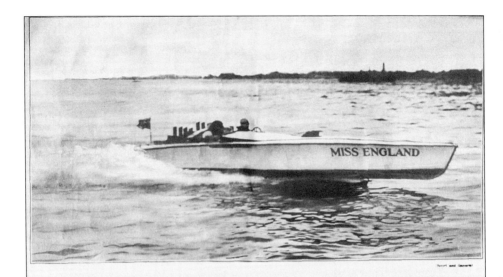

# SIR CHARLES WAKEFIELD'S
# "MISS ENGLAND"
# ON VIEW

# BOOKING HALL
# CHARING
# CROSS STATION

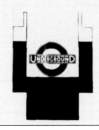

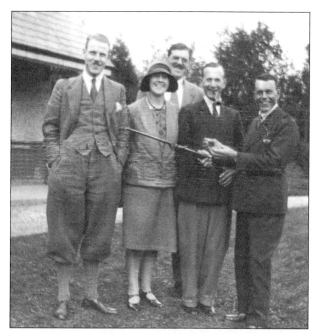

The design team: Lovell, Scovell, Mr and Mrs Fred Cooper and Michael Willcocks at Cooper's home in Hythe *(Michael Willcocks)*

The poster on the facing page, reproduced from a rare original, reflected the high level of public interest in the *Miss England* project *(Author's collection)*

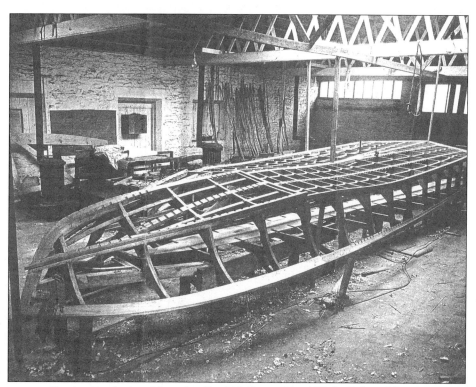

Construction begins at Saunders-Roe Ltd, Cowes, Isle of Wight *(Beken of Cowes)*

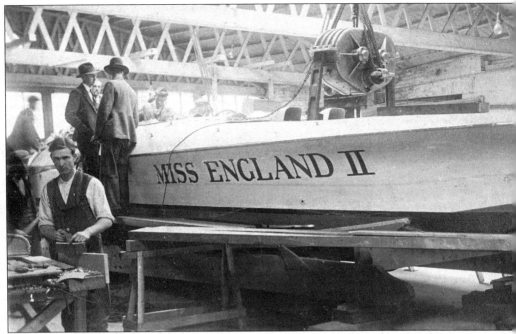

The building team. Notice gearbox hanging from crane *(The Motorboat Museum)*

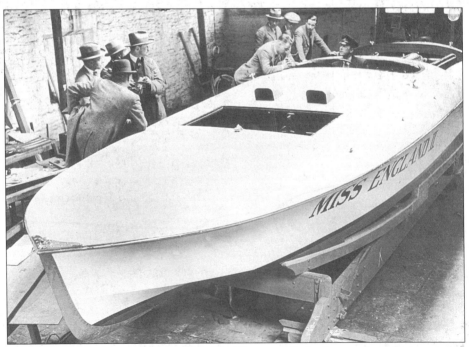

The Gentlemen of the Press interview Segrave as the boat nears completion
*(The Motorboat Museum)*

(Scotty received the following cable from Daytona Beach, Miami, Florida: "Mile timed today at 78 on 3/4 throttle. Boat ran dead horizontal, handles beautifully, no wash. Hull simply wonderful. Motor wonderful. Congratulations – Segrave.")

Barrett continues:

"After a successful trial run at Daytona Beach, Segrave shipped his boat to Miami Beach. He knew that if he could at least make a showing of this contest he'd have little difficulty in getting financial backing from Lord Wakefield for a future Harmsworth boat. He discussed the possibility with Wood and the American agreed that they should stage a close race. Wood was extremely anxious for Segrave to play an important role in Harmsworth competition.

"Segrave had a strong vivid stripe of the dare-devil in him. Before the race he asked Wood for the pole position. Wood said 'That's dangerous sir. My boat is faster. When I cut in on you you'll have to take my wash.' Segrave answered, 'I'll take the chance'. He was given pole position. When Wood cut across Segrave's bow the solid spray of *Miss America VII* struck Segrave full in the face. For a few desperate seconds Segrave didn't know what had happened.

"*Miss America VII* had been in the south for some time and the salt water had eaten away the steering cable, unbeknown to the Wood crew. The two boats made a beautiful start. The dark mahogany hull of the *Miss America* contrasted with the pure white hull of *Miss England*. The race was over a twelve-mile course and although *Miss America VII* led *Miss England* on the first turn, on making that turn the steering cable let go and Wood was unable to proceed.

"The news was flashed over the world that at last a British boat had beaten Gar Wood in a championship race. The rules governing this particular event were set up by the American Powerboat Association on what is known as a point system; and all the British boat had to do in the second heat was to finish to gain one more point than the American boat which did not finish the first heat. Segrave finished the second heat and won the race even though Gar Wood lapped him three times."

The following day, *Miss England* averaged 91.91mph over six sprints which although not enough for a new record, did show Gar Wood that the British were not far behind him. The day after that, Wood went out to reassure himself but was only able to clock a new average of 93.12mph, just under 0.3mph faster than his old mark. Segrave returned home to a hero's welcome in Southampton and again in London. A grateful King George V conferred a knighthood upon the sportsman who held the nation's honour in his hands.

Later that summer, Sir Henry Segrave took *Miss England* out to Venice for a return match against the *Miss America* team. The Duke of Spoletto, cousin of King Victor Immanuel, was in charge of the regatta. Gar Wood sent his *VII* over to the Lido with his brother Phil but, far from taking his revenge, in the race for the Prince of Italy's Cup, *Miss America VII* hit *Miss England's* wash with such impact that both Phil and riding mechanic Orlin Johnson were flicked into the water. The *VII* was a write-off and, following mouth-to-mouth resuscitation, Gar Wood's ever-faithful riding mechanic Johnson was taken to recover in an Italian hospital.

By the end of the 1929 season, Segrave and Scott-Paine had successfully piloted *Miss England* to win the International German and European Championship races among a total of eight motorboat victories. They had set up a new record for single-engined hydroplanes at 92.8mph. But with that last record, *Miss England* had reached the limit of her 930hp Napier aero-engine. Lord Wakefield donated *Miss England* to the Science Museum in London.

Segrave's 1929 *Miss England* victory had opened the door to British trade – sowing the seed for a new export market in motorboats and marine engines, that continues today. America was already in the lead with her network of over one thousand islands interconnected by lakes and rivers promoting the development of powerboating both with inboard runabouts or outboard engines. Great Britain was doing a moderate trade in motorboats. To boost that trade into foreign markets, to advertise the product, this needed a great and public adventure.

By October 1929, Sir Henry Segrave was living with his wife, Doris, in a large country-house called 'Warren End' on Kingston Hill, Surrey. At the end of their garden, there was a small wooden house with a thatched roof, inside which was Segrave's model railway. Its walls were 'rimmed' with a series of rails, at one point six lines wide. There were two stations, model

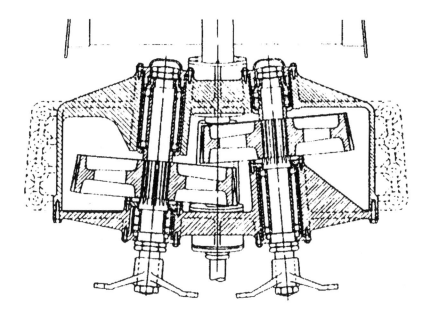

Gearbox of *Miss England II*

railwaymen, passengers, trains, signals and tracks. Segrave himself had taken some fourteen years to make practically everything himself and was particularly proud of that achievement.

As far as business went, Sir Henry was considerably involved – directorships in three companies and writing for various journals. He had also written a popular autobiography called 'The Lure of Speed'. He was involved with the design work of a multi-gadget, luxury sports car called the Hillman 'Segrave' and, as aviation adviser to the Aircraft Investment Corporation, he had been involved in the design and development of a high-speed four-seat twin-engined monoplane landplane of wooden construction, the Saunders-Roe A22 Segrave Meteor.

As an Imperialist, Sir Henry believed that, "The only bright ray for the economic future of our Empire lies with the United Empire party." As for the future of motorboat building in Britain, for Segrave – and indeed for Lord Wakefield – the only way ahead was to build a second boat, *Miss England II*, with which he could successfully challenge Gar Wood.

The concept of the new boat with which Segrave began to experiment, using toy boats, was the idea that instead of building a boat and getting the engines into it, he would take the engines and the gearbox, then build the sub-frame around them – a kind of car chassis concept applied to motorboats.

In his initial efforts, he was helped by an old friend, Bill Guinness, a member of the fabulously wealthy Dublin brewery dynasty. But when it got to a certain stage, the two amateurs handed over – not to Scott-Paine but to Fred Cooper. Cooper had been so embittered at Scott-Paine's claiming that only he had designed *Miss England I* that he resigned from the yard and set up on his own at 'Verulam'. He recruited two apprentices from the J.S. White boatyard, Bob Lovell and Tom Scovell, to help him with the detailed layout drawings of Segrave's new hydroplane.

Fred Cooper's wife Dolly later recalled, "We were living out on the edge of the New Forest at the time, and they worked into the early hours. The calculations they did were simply staggering. He spent a week doing the calculations for the gearbox alone. It was work, work, work all the time. We often used to have to phone up the post-mistress at Hythe and say, 'Would you please hold up the Post – Mr Cooper's on his way with some more drawings.' The panic was terrible!"

# 5

## The Bomb in the Eggshell

With the marine architects at work, the search began for two engines that would give Segrave the power he needed. At first he had considered using a pair of the latest 1,320hp boosted Napier Lion engines. But several months before, Segrave had taken His Royal Highness Edward, the Prince of Wales up in his private plane to watch the Schneider Trophy Air Race take place over Southampton Waters and Spithead. Together they had seen Flying Office H.R.D. Waghorn win the Trophy in a Supermarine Rolls-Royce S6 racing seaplane powered by the supercharged 12-cylinder 'R'-type engine, developing 1,800hp.

The story behind this engine is no ordinary one and has become legendary in British aero-engineering history. When the Air Ministry had asked Rolls-Royce to produce an aero-engine to power the new Supermarine S6 seaplane for the 1929 contest, there had been little time to come up with a totally original powerplant.

In October 1928, three of the company's technical staff – designer A.J. Rowledge with E.W. Hives of the Experimental Department and his assistant Lovesey – went down to see Sir Henry Royce at his home and headquarters at West Wittering. They found him enthusiastic. It was a bright autumn morning and Royce suggested a stroll along the beach. As they walked, the firm's co-founder and engineering genius pointed out the local places of interest. But Royce, who walked with a stick, soon tired. "Let's find a sheltered spot," he said, "and have a talk." Seated on the sand dunes against a groyne, Royce sketched the rough outline of a racing engine in the sand with his stick. Each man was asked his opinion in turn, the sand was raked over and adjustments made. The key to the engine was simplicity. "I invent nothing," was Royce's philosophy, "inventors go broke."

Like the Rolls-Royce Kestrel and Buzzard aero-engines, the new racing engine would have only 12 cylinders and much of it would be built of a new aluminium alloy (Hiduminium RR50). The secret of increased power would lie in supercharging. The power of an engine depends on the mass of air it can consume in a given time and a supercharger provides a means of getting additional air through an engine of given size and capacity.

Royce eventually guaranteed to produce en engine of around 1,500 horse-power – and maybe 1,800 horse-power. The 'R' (for Racing) engine was modified to ensure better streamlining. Around this, Supermarine Aviation's talented aircraft designer, R. J. Mitchell (later famous for the Spitfire fighter plane) could begin to sketch out the lines for the S6 racing seaplane. With the increased engine size and consumption, both floats must now be used as fuel tanks. By May 1929, the first 'R' engines were assembled by Rolls-Royce at their Derby works. On 14th May, running at 2,750 rpm, engine 'R1' gave 1,545 brake horse-power, but after only fifteen minutes parts began to fail. By 5th July, engine R7 managed an increased 1,718bhp for a long period.

Throughout that summer, the test-beds at Derby reverberated with the sound of the world's most powerful racing aero-engine – and of the auxiliary engines that were an integral part of the test rig. There were three of these, all 600hp Kestrels. Two were driving fans, one to cool the engine crankcase and the other to disperse the fumes that filled the test-house. The third auxiliary engine drove a special fan, which provided an airflow into the forward-facing air intake of up to 380mph, simulating the conditions that would be encountered in flight.

When the wind was in a prevailing direction, the noise of these four engines going full blast could be heard all over Derby. The sound acted as a barometer of progress. When the new engine ran sweetly there was optimism. When it remained silent for long periods there was despair. The target for the Rolls-Royce technicians was one hour's run of a proof engine at maximum speed and boost. On thirteen occasions one of this first batch of 'R'-engines broke down before the hour was up. But on 27th July, less than six weeks before the race and thanks to a special aviation fuel mixture developed by F.R. Banks to prevent pre-ignition problems, the hour target was met and soon a satisfactory life of 100 minutes at 1,850hp had been achieved. The proved 'R' type was transported to Supermarine Aviation Company at Woolston, Southampton.

Rolls-Royce's programme paid off. Not only did Flying Officer Waghorn pilot his S6 seaplane to a victorious 328mph average for the seven laps – so defending the Schneider Trophy for Great Britain – but also, on 12th September, Squadron Leader A.H. Orlebar used the R-engined S6 seaplane to seize the World Air Speed Record at 357.7mph. With the daring idea that two of these 'R' types in one boat would give him the speed he was looking for, Segrave used his influence to persuade those in power to contract to build a pair to the order of Lord Wakefield. These were numbered R17 and R19. Of these two, R17 was probably the rarest of all R-types for it was the only engine built as a left-hand tractor, in other words it spun the other way. This was to eliminate the problem of matching engine speeds in a twin-engined craft.

# 6

# The Riding Mechanics

With the design of the boat about to pass on to its construction by Saunders-Roe of Cowes, on the Isle of Wight, Segrave, who had always used a riding mechanic with *Miss England I*, began to ask around for a mate. Fred Cooper suggested an engineer called Willcocks as one possibility. Michael J. Willcocks was born in Clevedon, Somerset in 1884. He recalled: "My father was a seafaring man, and as a child I can remember being taken out in a gale of wind. I was always keen on boats, but I was frightfully keen on aeroplanes. I was building my own full-size glider and I'd hoped to install a twin-cylinder horizontal-post engine, then the First World War intervened. But I did get two hops. I cycled down to Larkshill and had a spin with Bendall, the instructor-pilot at the Bristol School of Aviation.

"Although people don't realise it, it was very difficult to get into anything in the 1914 war. I couldn't get into anything because I was undersize – I'm only 4ft 4 ins. So I went to Coventry Technical College, where I trained as an engineer on gauge work, and from there to London, then on to Hayes at the aero-engine factory. I then re-applied to go into the Air Force.

"After waiting a week at Brooke Street, I was told to go down and see Commander O'Connor at the Admiralty, where I was taken on straightaway as Chief Motor Mechanic on hydroplanes.

"After the War, Sir Alfred Bailey was living over here at Bristol. There were a lot of 'Motor Boat' magazines, which had been chucked away over the sea wall, because somebody local had bought the place and had thrown these copies away. In these I saw that Segrave was racing against Gordon Selfridge and a few others on the Thames.

"So I wrote to the Johnson outboard engine people for the design of a single-step hydroplane with a twin-cylinder Johnson engine. I called my boat *Osea I*. Then, in about 1927, I joined with several others in forming an Outboard Racing Club at Bristol. I even won a cup for driving an outboard motorboat across the treacherous waters of the Bristol Channel and back. After that I got a bigger Johnson engine and raced in both Wales and along the south coast.

"Before competing at the 'Daily Mirror' outboard race at Hythe, Hants, two of the lads and myself saw *Miss England I* at the British Powerboat Company, just as she was being packed ready to go to the Venice Lido. I knew she was designed by Fred Cooper and shortly after, I asked Fred to design a boat for me to try and break the Cowes Sea Class Record, using a Douglas dirt-track engine. I never finished this because in one of my letters to Fred I'd said 'I notice you're designing the big one, Number *II*. If you want a watchman or store-keeper on the job, I'd like to go. I haven't had a holiday for years and as long as expenses are paid, I'd be only too pleased.' Cooper wrote back, 'If you would like to ride as mate to Sir Henry, I can fix an appointment for you in London.'

"I went to see Segrave at the offices of Blue Circle Cement, whose Managing Director, Andrew Holt, was a close friend of Segrave's. I went up by train. I stuck my head out of the window to get an idea as to whether I could possibly stand up to the speed, with no windscreen or anything. I've got a very small nose and at high speed my nose closes in and I've a job to breathe. I was pretty nervous on that journey.

"I had been very, very impressed by Segrave's Land Speed Record successes. What influenced me as much as anything was Segrave's speech when he came back from America. He said 'I'm sure Lord Wakefield and Andrew Holt will be very annoyed with me for mentioning that this would have been impossible but for their help.' I admired him no end for that.

"I was taken in to this office and Segrave came in. He was wearing an ordinary lounge suit, not a City Waller's suit. My first impression was of his height, and that the sides of his hair were a bit long and needed cutting. I noticed his blue eyes very quickly. He had a very clean and very mobile face, very intelligent-looking. He looked at me straight in the eyes, summing me

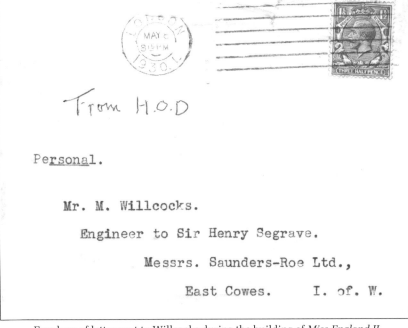

Envelope of letter sent to Willcocks during the building of *Miss England II*

up. I looked back at him. He had a very strong, penetrating voice.

"You would like to go on this boat?"

"Yes sir."

"Why do you want to go?"

"I hate the godamm Yanks winning all the races."

"Well you realise that this is going to be no joy-ride."

"Yes."

"If anything happens, seriously happens, at the speeds we hope to go, there will be no-one left alive."

"I think I realise that sir. But in any case, if I go, I think my parents would like anything that's left sent back to Clevedon."

"Yes, that could be arranged. Now, how much do you want to do the job?"

"Nothing. I can't afford to pay my own expenses. I haven't much money. We're only a small business."

"I won't have anyone victimised. You must have something. How about £4 10 shillings a week and expenses?"

"Whatever you say, sir."

"I'll want you to spend a week at Windermere and three

weeks in the States. We shall race at Detroit, then go and run on the river at Toronto at the same time as the Canadian National Exhibition. I won't accept your decision now. Go home and think about it for a week. At Miami, *Miss England I*'s oil-cooler packed up. Englishmen specialise. An American called Sig Haugdahl went up in the town and bought a water geezer ... from this he built an oil cooler which is in the boat to this day. This is the type of man I require. Think it over. When you've made up your mind, if you say no, I shan't think any the less of you. If you say yes, I expect you to stay with the job to the end."

"The interview had lasted about quarter-of-an-hour. He was very nice, charming. I felt an absolute trust. I could never conceive anything going wrong with Segrave driving."

Willcocks returned by train to his Clevedon home.

"That was the worst week I had spent, churning it over in my mind. Whether I had enough experience, whether I could back up the job. Although I could show a pretty good engineering experience, it worried me that I'd never seen a Schneider Trophy engine and I didn't know anything about water-cooling systems. When Sir Henry had said he would want someone who could replace anything that went wrong, that was a big proposition. It was a challenge. I didn't know whether I had enough guts to do it.

"I didn't tell my girlfriend about it. But I told my parents, my brothers and sisters. I think my mother was worried. She realised the danger, although she never gave out what she was feeling. My father was pleased. My brothers were delighted. I told Dr Renton, Chairman of the local Rugby Club and he said, 'You go, my boy. You're all right.'

"I went to see the family doctor and asked to be thoroughly overhauled. If there was anything wrong, he must tell me. He said, 'Well, you are on the verge of a breakdown physically because you haven't had a holiday for donkey's years. But otherwise I see no medical reasons to hold you back.'"

At the end of the week, Willcocks wrote to Segrave stating that he would like to go and that he accepted the conditions. Segrave wrote back:

"I should be obliged if you'd go to Cowes and see the installation because the one who's going to look after it, should see it installed. I would also like you to keep an eye on the building of the Meteor monoplane."

A fortnight later Willcocks had packed his suitcase, telling his girlfriend Helen that he was going away for a long holiday.

"The worry was that if I was sacked through being incompetent, it would react on the business and because I was not absolutely confident that I knew enough to do the job, I gave the Press the false name of 'Michael Wilson, from a garage on the south coast.'"

The speedboat was being built in a small shed at Saunders-Roe's Cornubia Works on East Cowes. To preserve the utmost secrecy, a guard was mounted day and night. Other parts were being put together at three different sites – J. Samuel White Ltd. had also subcontracted certain parts, whilst some work was being done at Parsons Ltd., a big garage in Southampton. Willcocks made a stiff board chart for all the pieces and visited each of the four local sites twice a day. He walked the twelve miles so as to improve his physical fitness in readiness for crewing the hydroplane. He would ring Fred Cooper every morning and give him a progress report.

"As the bits came in, I checked them. For example, I checked the propshaft by putting it on some V-blocks that were strapped to a long table. Rotating the shaft, I found it was an inch and a quarter out of true. Fred Cooper came over and checked this with Mr Piper at the works.

"I said 'If anything goes wrong, my bottom is not very far from that. I don't feel very happy about it.' So they condemned that one, and Thornycrofts supplied a new one which was truer."

So that the speedboat would be ready for her official launching on Windermere in the English Lake District the following June, the pressure was considerable; Segrave described it as 'eight and a half months of concentrated work, brain fag and fatigue.'

Fred Cooper rang Willcocks one morning, some fourteen days before the projected transport of the boat to Windermere. He was concerned that, of the seven propellers ordered, none had yet been finished. Willcocks went to see the foreman who was doing this forging only to be told that the new power hammer ordered express for this purpose had not been delivered. However, one propeller had been forged and was in the finishing shop for grinding and polishing. Willcocks said: "I explained the urgency to millwright foreman Ted Smith. He replied that he would grind the forging himself. At midday I had completed my first daily round of inspection when a message came that the grinding wheel had burst and killed Ted Smith. Normally, he would have been protected by a hood around the grinding wheel but he had taken this off to give the propeller clearance and was doing it by hand when the wheel had jammed and exploded in his face. It shook me to the core, because I felt directly responsible. I was the one who'd said it was urgent."

Rolls-Royce wanted to obtain a complete record of the performance of the 'R'-type engines, so they asked Segrave to take a second riding mechanic – one for each engine. Although this had not been in the original plan, it was decided that this might be a good idea. The 31-year-old engineer selected was one of Rolls-Royce's most brilliant engineers.

Percival Victor Conrad Halliwell was born in 1899 at Portishead, Somerset, the son of an insurance broker. From the Fairfield School in Bristol, in 1915 and at only sixteen years old, Vic Halliwell obtained a Scholarship to the University of Bristol. In 1917 he left the Engineering Faculty to join the Royal Flying Corps. He was soon promoted from Second to First Class Air Mechanic, eventually obtaining a commission as a lieutenant and second officer in the newly formed RAF. On the Armistice he returned to Bristol University, specialising in automobile engineering and graduating as Bachelor of Science, still aged only 21. From December 1920 until May 1921, Halliwell was working in the 'Wave Transmission' drawing office of W.H. Dorman and Co. Ltd, international combustion engine specialists in Stafford. He worked on the design of a complete powerplant, as well as detailing the building up a general arrangement of drawings. His curriculum vitae in 1923 stated that he was a Consulting Automobile Engineer, also engaged in research work under Professor Morgan in the Automobile Laboratory of Bristol University.

In 1925, Halliwell obtained a job at Rolls-Royce in the aero-engine department. Three years later he joined the team in developing the 'R'-type engine. Following the Schneider

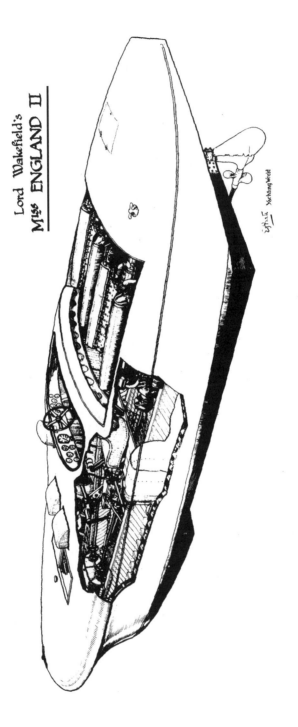

E.J. Pratt's superb cutaway drawings regularly enriched the pages of the yachting press *(Quadrant Picture Library)*

Trophy victory, Halliwell soon became involved in the *Miss England II* venture. Originally, he was responsible for developing both engines and a water-cooling system – before taking these down to the Isle of Wight for installation in the boat. In so far as acting as a riding mechanic in potentially the world's fastest speedboat, Halliwell decided not to tell his family. Several years before, a brother had been drowned in the Thames and this had severely distressed his mother. He therefore did not want to cause her unnecessary anxiety.

Willcocks recalled his first meeting with his future crew mate. "When I saw him at Southampton's West Quay, I realised that we had already met. I'd filled up a works Rolls-Royce car for him at our Clevedon Garage. He'd been on his way from his Portishead family home bound for the Schneider Trophy contest.

"I said 'D'you know, I am pleased to see you. We thought we were going to get one of those snotty-nosed Naval Officers!'

"I liked Halliwell. He was a very nice chap, married with an infant son. But I felt he was much too frail for the job. Segrave was tall, but with broad shoulders he was strong. Halliwell was tall but academic-looking."

\* \* \* \* \*

A 'Daily Mirror' reporter-friend of Segrave's was soon allowed to see the half-finished craft in Cowes. He wrote of how he found Segrave sitting on the edge of the cockpit, lost in profound thought. "Hello, come up the ladder and have a good look at her. Isn't she fine?" he is reported to have said. It was a typical Segrave trait that machines, no matter for what element, had to be the latest, biggest, strongest, fastest or some other superlative. And *Miss England II* was certainly proof of it. She was described as 'a floating experiment' and 'like cramming a bomb into an eggshell'. Her strength was her most important aspect.

"Imagine, then, this hull," the reporter wrote, "not skimming the surface of soft water, but bumping across a ploughed field at 100mph and some conception of the necessary strength can be arrived at."

Her hull had been covered with three 'skins' – two diagonal and one longitudinal with fabric and mariner glue between the surfaces. These 'skins' were made out of steel, then Duralmin, then Honduras mahogany. As well as this, twin engine bearers for each engine, not less than 14 inches deep ran from aft to forward, closing into the support gearbox. These were made from Canadian rock elm and braced with pitch pine.

As a one-step hydroplane, her step had been fixed on afterwards by over eighty specially-made, stainless steel nuts and bolts and was about the size of a suburban garage door. The hull bottom had been painted entirely black, polished with powdered graphite and embedded in special liquid dressing. Her sides had been painted white gloss. *Miss England II* had been stencilled on both sides of her bows in red letters, shaded black. Her deck was of canvas, coloured very light grey. In overall design, she as very similar to her elder sister except for a special Vee- or ducktail-shaped stern to minimise drag and a deep, flat forward deck. Her measurements were 38 feet 6 inches long, and 10 feet 6 inches extreme width.

The 'bomb' that was crammed into this 'eggshell' was even more revolutionary for its time. Instead of the two Rolls-Royce engines having two gearboxes and two propellers (or screws), they both drove forward at 2,900 revolutions per minute (rpm) into each side of only *one* gearbox, the largest of its kind ever produced, oil-cooled, and with special gear wheels cut by the E.N.V. Engineering Company. Almost always, the job of a gearbox in a boat is to *reduce* the number of rpm going back to the propeller to give the screw greater grip as it spins through the water. But with *Miss England II*, it was a case of multiplying the revs no less than four times, so that the submerged propeller would spin at the rate of 12,550 to 13,000rpm.

Such a daring technical approach was unprecedented in the history of marine engineering. In consequence the propeller shaft was only $1\frac{5}{8}$ inches in diameter, but of a solid steel tensile strength of 120 tons per square inch. The bow and stern rudders, connected to the drop arm of the steering column had been carved from plates of 100-ton, air-hardening nickel chrome steel.

The single submerged propeller would have to be extremely strong not only because of the speeds at which it would be spinning, but also because it would have to be so small. This size factor was due to the attempt to avoid 'torque'. Torque is created when, instead of the screw rotating around the boat, the

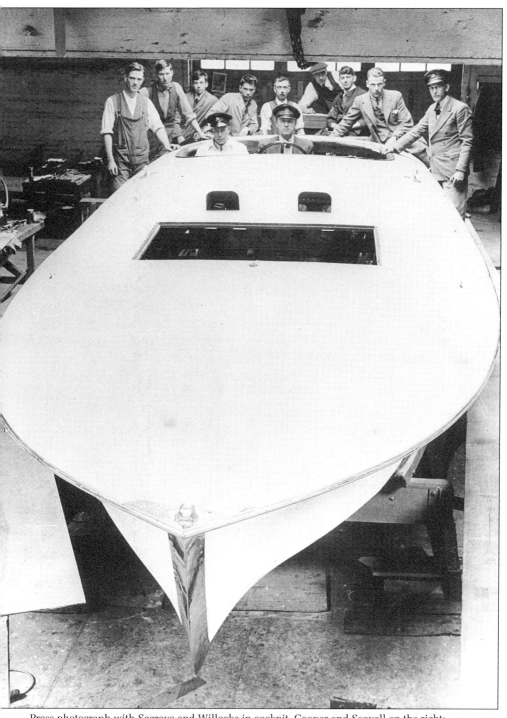

Press photograph with Segrave and Willocks in cockpit, Cooper and Scovell on the right; Fred Goatley and Saunders-Roe team around the stern *(Author's collection)*

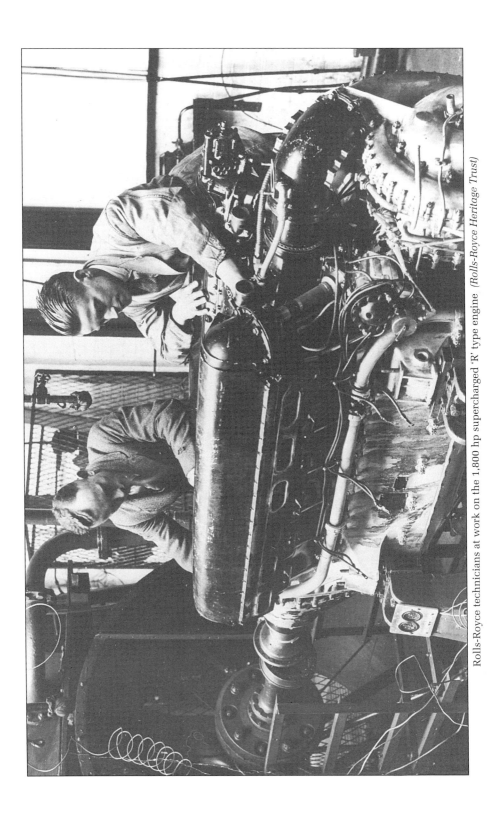

Rolls-Royce technicians at work on the 1,800 hp supercharged 'R' type engine *(Rolls-Royce Heritage Trust)*

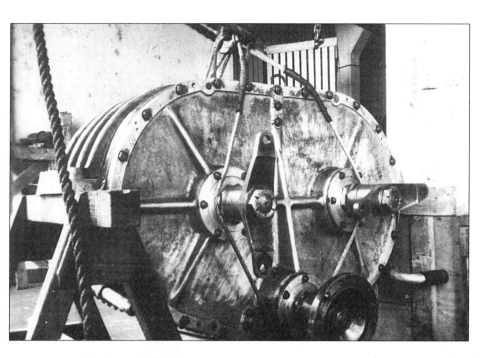

The gearbox was the largest of its kind ever produced, with special gear wheels cut by the E.N.V. Engineering Company *(Michael Willcocks)*

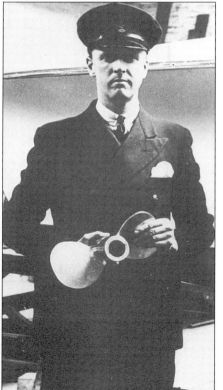

Segrave is shown holding the crucial two-bladed propeller *(Author's collection)*

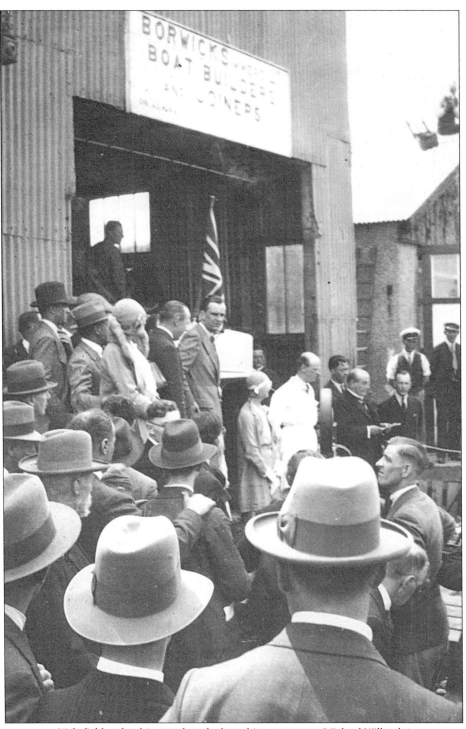

Wakefield makes his speech at the launching ceremony *(Michael Willcocks)*

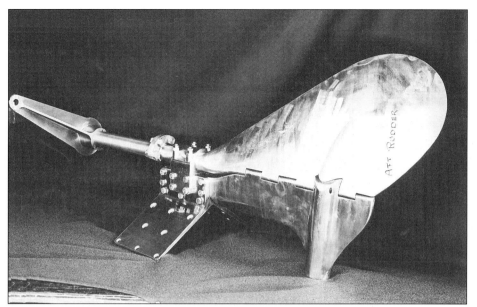

*Miss England II* had both fore and aft rudders, carved from plates of 100-ton air-hardening nickel chrome steel. This is the aft rudder *(Author's collection)*

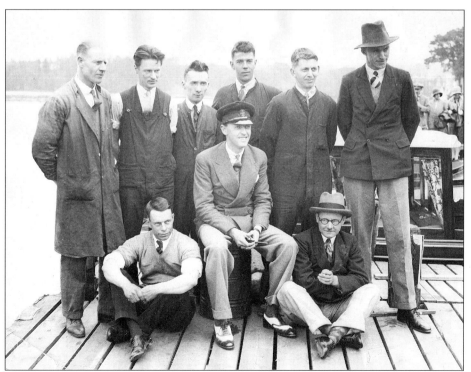

The team on the jetty at Bowness-on-Windermere. Willcocks seated, Halliwell in the trilby hat *(Author's collection)*

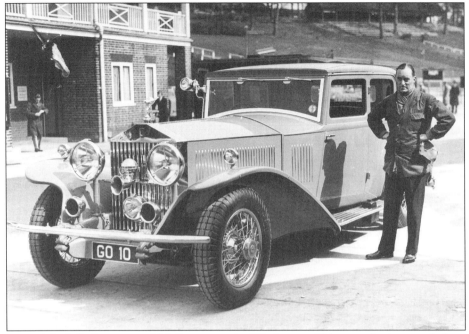

One of the Rolls-Royce cars which Segrave used at Windermere. This example photographed at Brooklands with Sir Malcolm Campbell, his major rival *(Rolls-Royce Heritage Trust)*

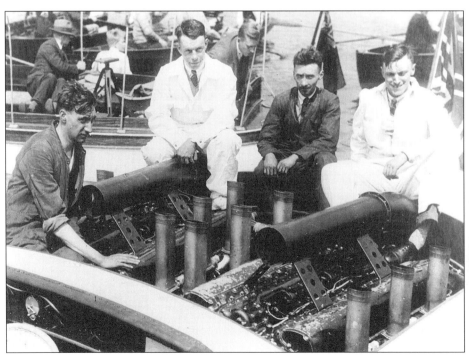

Willcocks and Halliwell astride 3,600 horsepower! *(Author's collection)*

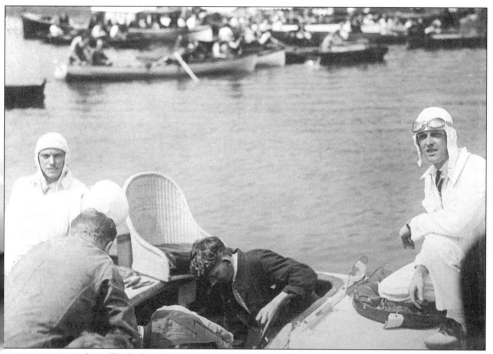

Sound-muffler helmets on, prior to a trial run. Note the lightweight wicker seat
*(Author's collection)*

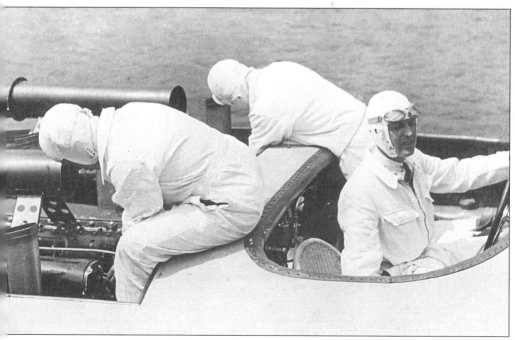

On your marks for a trial run. Get set to fire up engines *(Victor Halliwell)*

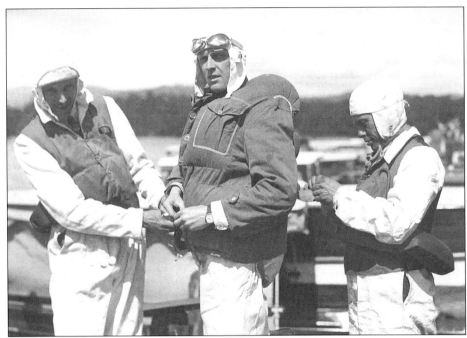

The lifejackets were made from inadequate padded reindeer hair. The steel versions were late in delivery *(Quadrant Picture Library)*

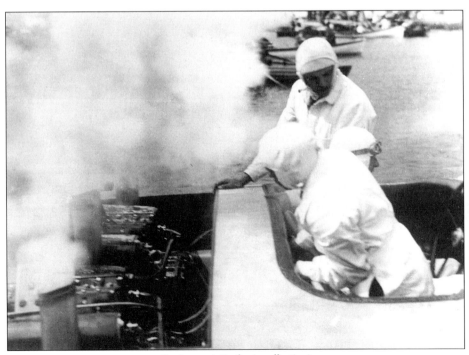

Engines go! *(Author's collection)*

boat is trying to rotate around the screw. Segrave and Cooper had specified no less than seven propellers with different pitches and diameters – but all quite small – to try to cope with this problem.

Finally, the cockpit itself. Piloting *Miss England II* was going to be like driving *two* racing cars at the same time: except for the steering wheel, there were two of everything. Two throttles, two clutches, two tachometers, four engine switches (two for the starter motors and two for the main aero-unit), two engine water temperature gauges, two stern tube temperature gauges, two gearbox water temperature gauges, two engine oil pressure gauges, two engine oil temperature gauges, and so on. All in all, this added up to over thirty instruments – including the steering wheel – to control. As yet, the seats had not been fitted, not to mention numerous other details, several of which are mentioned above.

\* \* \* \* \*

So much for the machine, but what about the man? In 1930 Henry Segrave was 34-years-old. Physically he was tall, slenderly built, with piercing deep-set blue eyes, well set in his hawk-like face, and reddish but prematurely balding hair. Although fit and strong, very active and full of energy, when under considerable strain, he would limp from pain caused by his left ankle, part of which was artificially supported by silver plates fitted after a wartime plane crash. Often his public-school accent betrayed what was at the time considered as slight Americanese with words such as 'fine' – a complementary expression he often used.

In terms of personality, Segrave was the quietest and least assuming of gentlemen. He was very calm and cool and could not be pushed into anything he did not want to do. He would not take a risk unless it was a calculated risk. He had considerable charm, impeccable manners and was very kindly disposed and gentle towards women. No novice ever asked help or information from him without obtaining it. Segrave was famous for the generosity he showed to others, sincere in his praise of their success, making light of his own.

The worst they ever found to say against him was that he could put up a good bluff and that he was a showman ... and those who called his bluff always found that he held a stronger hand than his bluff ever suggested. Those who thought he was making a show with insufficient backing, found that he was probably making a show of some minor thing to distract attention from something more important, which he was holding in reserve.

# 7

# Windermere

Set in the north-west of England, between Lancashire and Westmorland, Windermere's majestic 10-mile length makes it the largest natural lake in the country. The first paddle steamer had appeared on this lake in 1845, the first motorboat in 1898 and the first motorboat racing in 1923/24. *Miss England II*, far from finished, left her boatyard at East Cowes on the morning of Thursday 29th May 1930. After an uneventful crossing of the Solent by steamer, she was hoisted onto the tyre-and-straw bale supports of the eight-wheel Scammell lorry that was to take her unruly size along a specially mapped route up to the banks of Windermere.

Although the weight of the hydroplane was only 4.5 tons, the laden weight of the lorry was 19 tons. It would be a slow journey. *Miss England II* was covered only in a Union Jack tarpaulin but, as Britain had been enjoying an extraordinarily fine summer, such a covering was considered ample. This was the beginning of a journey that would take her up to Windermere for an attempt on the Water Speed Record, then to challenge Gar Wood for the Harmsworth Trophy races at Detroit, and from there on to the Canadian National Exhibition at Toronto.

On her way up the Great North Road, the British speedboat pilot Betty Carstairs drew alongside the lorry in her Bentley and shouted up to Willcocks, "Witness the first and last time that I'll pass *Miss England II*!" Miss Carstairs was planning to travel out to Detroit with a couple of her Napier aero-engined speedboats called *Estelle* – and joined by the *Miss England II* team, give Commodore Gar Wood, the defending Harmsworth Trophy champion 'a run for his money'.

With efficiency typical of a Segrave venture, accommodation and course organisation had already been arranged several months previously. *Miss England II* and her tender-boat, *Miss London* – also Segrave's private runabout – were to have both 'dry' and 'wet' docks at 'Messrs Borwicks Ltd, Boatbuilders and Joiners' on the shores of Bowness Bay. Borwicks had even rigged a special crane with timbers, girders and a chain, with which *Miss England II*'s considerable weight could be lifted from her Scammell and into her dry dock. A day-and-night guard had been arranged with the local constabulary.

Accommodation for Segrave's party, Sir Charles Wakefield's party – including several Castrol representatives – Fred Cooper and the team from Cowes, Vic Halliwell and the team from Derby, had been arranged all over Bowness. The nearest large hotel, booked to overflowing, was by a coincidence called 'The Old England Hotel'. Its proprietor was Mr Roger Bownass.

In a letter dated 14$^{th}$ April, Segrave wrote to Mr Bownass:

"Lady Segrave also wishes to bring a small lap dog. I take it there would be no objection to this if we have a sitting room – the dog is thoroughly well trained and would never be seen anyway."

Segrave had also informed the members of the Windermere Town Council of the brief running time of the 'R'-type engines: "I do not anticipate that during the whole of my stay the boat will be on the waters of the lake for a longer running period than five hours and this may be shortened if initial runs prove satisfactory."

The Windermere Council had given its full permission for the use of the Lake. Segrave should regain the World Record for Britain on British waters. The Windermere Motor Boat Racing Club considered it an honour to give such a venture its fullest co-operation: Major Harold Pattinson, its Chairman, did everything in his power to see that both course organisation, traffic control on both land and water, and the trials themselves should run smoothly.

On the afternoon of June 1$^{st}$, after a seven-hour journey, the Segraves arrived at the parking ground opposite Borwicks in a 44 horsepower Rolls-Royce Phantom, the louvres of its jet-black sports car body elegantly picked out in cream. On the front bumper were displayed the badges of eleven motor clubs of different nationalities. Peach, his chauffeur, accompanied him in a 26 horsepower Rolls with eight entirely different badges on its bumper. Minutes after inspecting *Miss England II*, Segrave went out for a spin in *Miss London* with Fred Cooper and Major Pattinson to inspect the course. This was to be on the west side of the lake, about a quarter of a mile from the shore, where a clear run of about four miles of lake was available for acceleration and deceleration. Large pyramid-shaped buoys painted in black and white stripes marked the Measured Nautical Mile. The Signalling Corps was to assist Colonel Lindsay Lloyd and George Reynolds, the official Royal Automobile Club timekeepers, with their chronometers. There were four telephones for land use, one at each end of the course, and one at each end of the Measured Mile. Segrave returned, thanking and congratulating Course Marshall Pattinson on his work.

Launching was at noon on Thursday – in four days' time. The course was ready, but the hydroplane was not. Segrave – and Peach, his chauffeur – rolled up their sleeves. It was summertime – Windermere was only getting dark at around 10 o'clock in the evening and sunrise came in the early hours. Segrave talked of the final preparations: "We have had about nine fellows voluntarily working through two and a half whole nights without any rest at all, only leaving the boathouse to snatch a hurried meal." There was no question of overtime pay, just everyone working until the job was finished. Segrave was once heard to say to Cooper, 'How about some food Fred?' 'Excellent idea!' came the response – though on Wednesday night they paused – 'wondering' in Segrave's words, 'just what would go wrong.'

The following morning, just to check they were running well, Segrave gave his engines a land test, little expecting that one of the clutches would seize. Although this caused some anxiety among the crew, it was decided that very little could be done in the short time remaining to them. There were still other little matters to be seen to: the wicker-work seats had not been put in yet.

Although it was Ascot week and the Aldershot Tattoo was on, the turnout on and around Windermere as it neared midday, had to be seen to be believed – thousands of people and an estimated fleet of no less than six hundred craft had gathered to get a closer view of what had been described as 'the £25,000 aristocrat of inland waterways', 'the white witch of Windermere' and 'the black-bottomed bombshell'.

TELEPHONE Nos { SOUTHAMPTON 4662 : LONDON. VICTORIA 2525

CODES:- A B C 5ᵀᴴ EDITION BENTLEY'S

TELEGRAMS { "MOTORS" SOUTHAMPTON.

LONDON OFFICE: 3. VICTORIA STREET, WESTMINSTER, S.W.I.

# THE PARSONS OIL ENGINE Cº. LTD.

## OIL & PETROL ENGINE BUILDERS.

CONTRACTORS TO THE
ADMIRALTY, WAR OFFICE, INDIA OFFICE,
CROWN AGENTS AND TO FOREIGN GOVERNMENTS.

MARINE SET.

STATIONARY SET.

Your Ref.

Our Ref. PES/EMB/WORKS DEPT.

### Town Quay Works,

# SOUTHAMPTON,

10th May, 1930.

Mr. Willcox,
   Messrs. Saunders-Roe Ltd.,
   "Miss England 11" Shed,
     COWES.

Dear Mr. Willcox,

       "MISS ENGLAND 11" STERN TUBE.

     We have made adjustments to the stern tube, and in order that you might have the opportunity of seeing how the aft bush fits thereto and the alignment of same, we have bushed down as you will notice to the size of the test shaft, and think you will agree that there is now perfect alignment.

     Part of the trouble was due to the **2.1/8"** bore tube which was found under size. This has been adjusted, and you will notice that the bush fits O.K. We have included the quickly made spanner for tightening the bush, so that you may remove same, and perhaps you might wish to forward this to Messrs. Goodrich for lining after removing the adaptors.

     On the other hand if you wish us to do so, it will mean returning this to us to be forwarded from here.

     We might add that had we retained the previous bush instead of forwarding it for lining prior to sending the tube to you, and used it in a similar manner as we have done now, the element of error would not have been introduced.

     Trusting that you will now be perfectly satisfied.

     Yours faithfully,

     THE PARSONS OIL ENGINE CO.LTD.

One of the many letters sent by suppliers of component parts *(Michael Willcocks)*

It was a field day for the Press. Cameramen ('still boys' and 'movie men') were dotted all over the place – on roofs, on launches, on the jetty and by the boathouse. Lord Wakefield and his party, including the Segraves, arrived – including Lord Brecknock and Atcherly, the Schneider Trophy winner and personal friend of Segrave. Wakefield began to speak into the microphone:

"It is my firm belief that scientific endeavour in the three fields of land, air and water should be encouraged to the fullest possible extent ..." During his short speech, Segrave later commented " ... if you could go behind the scenes with me you would have a very different thing on your minds."

Two Saunders-Roe employees, Henry Martin and Sidney Bowfield, were still screwing the seats into place. Michael Willcocks, having received the signal to clear decks, hurriedly closed and lifted Segrave's multi-compartment tool box. The spring lock did not lock as he lifted it and the contents – hundreds of small screws, nuts and bolts spilled onto the spotless deck. Frantically, 'Wilkie' cleared it up with a dustpan and brush.

"I christen you Miss England the Second," Wakefield declared and swung the champagne bottle at her bows. The boat moved forward, slid into the water and took up her position with ease and grace, whilst three lusty cheers rang out amidst continued clapping. Segrave, Cooper and Willcocks, in spotless white overalls, took up their positions in the cockpit and prepared to give the boat its first demonstration run. An aeroplane circled overhead whilst the adjustments were being made. The spectators' boats were approaching with daring familiarity. Two of the movie men's launches had come athwart *Miss England II*'s bows.

"For God's sake get out of the way! I have very little control at the start," Segrave shouted. The boats made way. Suddenly, out of the throat of the exhaust stacks, came a volley of smoke rings, there was a slight pause, then amidst clouds of smoke that followed came the typical subdued hum of the 'R'-type aero-engines starting up. As *Miss England II* moved out, the flotilla of spectators moved in. "If I had killed a few people," he recalled, "there would have been no end of a row."

Rather than risk swamping them in his wash, or even

running the smaller craft down, Segrave had to pilot her along at only 15mph. This proved fatal to the water-cooling system of a boat designed to function at higher speeds. And before he had even swerved out onto the course, before *Miss England II* had even travelled half a mile, steam was escaping from her port engine jacket in such a disconcerting manner that he turned her engines off at once. She was humiliatingly towed back to the jetty by a launch. Segrave had to face the Press: "We have discovered several minor details which need tuning up. During our short spin we went quite far enough to find out these minor points, such as leaks in the piping inside the boat et cetera." He added that *Miss England* might be ready by Tuesday – in five days' time.

At a huge VIP luncheon party at the Old England Hotel, Lord Wakefield said, "Today we have witnessed the beginning of a great adventure. A wonderful vessel has been launched which will carry within its comparatively frail frame the most power-ful machinery ever brought within so small a compass. It is to be piloted by a man who is not only a superb human machine but is also possessed of an astute and resourceful mind."

To those objecting to the noise from speedboats on the lake, Lord Howe asked them to be patient. "It is not to be an everyday affliction," he said. "We merely ask the people of Windermere for their co-operation as it is the only stretch of water in the British Isles suitable for the purpose."

Under the shadow of such an anti-climax, the return to hard work was inevitable. Due to the problem of the seizing clutch it was decided to delete the two clutches in place of two straight shafts installed in their place. As for water-cooling, it was decided to fit variable scoops to enable the by-pass valves to operate at any speed. Borwicks constructed new flow meters over the weekend.

During that weekend – Whitsun weekend – the crowds became so thick that even if *Miss England II* had been ready, she couldn't have gone out. Tension mounted. An elderly couple, wanting to have a peep at the boat, entered the boathouse without permission. One of the mechanics saw them and shouted, "Get out! You're not allowed in here!" Segrave, who happened to be out of sight of this mechanic, surprised him by shouting back, "And what d'you mean? These people have just as much right to come here as you have – standing there doing nothing!"

From then on, there was a roped walkway along which the public could pass, should they want to see the boat. According to Willcocks: "A little show was put on for the Movietone people. We had to walk alongside a temporary dockside and shake hands with Segrave. It seemed a bit stiff and artificial. When it came to my turn I grinned and said 'Do we qualify for star rating sir?' He laughed and said 'We certainly deserve it'."

Segrave the mechanic also found himself having to be Segrave the driver. The Windermere Motor Boat Racing Club, of which he had been elected an honorary member, was holding one of its weekend 'meets'. Segrave, international motor boat champion, after getting some practise in by figure-of-eighting *Miss London* around Bowness Bay, cruised her to an obviously sporting defeat against his fellow members, including several of their wives.

Meanwhile, Vic Halliwell had gone down to Derby to collect a new propeller from Rolls-Royce. During the post-mortem of the maiden run, it had been decided to fit a different propeller, because the one fitted had been found too small to spin at the very high revs it was meant to do. The prop situation down at Saunders-Roe on the Isle of Wight, had been rather desperate. Only a fortnight before the launching, a single screw had been forged and was in their finishing shop for grinding and polishing when seven more, with various pitches and diameters, were ordered by Segrave and Cooper. When the grinding wheel for that first prop disintegrated in foreman Ted Smith's face, with fatal results, it was decided to approach Rolls-Royce to see what they could come up with.

The result was the realisation of a revolutionary idea of design: a marine propeller using aircraft propeller principles. For the construction of this screw, a totally new technique was tried out. A solid billet of 'Stan Royal' high-speed steel, was supplied by the English Steel Corporation of Sheffield; instead of being forged, it was literally machined down to nine-tenths of its size. This left 100 inches for final machining after heat treatment, which involved intensive heating up to 840°C, then quenching in oil, then tempering by heating to 570°C and quenching in oil once more. This was done to give a tensile strength of 120 tons per square inch. The billet had weighed 170lb (77kg) and the finished propeller just 17lb (7.7kg). The prop was then polished so finely that it could cut the finger of the highly-skilled operator who carved it. When this prop was ready, it was immediately fixed to the rear part of the propshaft and this in turn was lashed to the side of Halliwell's 'works' Rolls-Royce and rushed up to Windermere for installation.

By Tuesday morning, *Miss England II* had been modified and her crew was mentally drilled for the first high speed run. With white racing overalls, red lifejackets (padded with special reindeer hair), and soft white helmets, Segrave, Willcocks and Halliwell climbed down into the cockpit. *Miss England II* was already in the water. The screws of her adjustable front step had been tightened, her sparking plugs changed, warm oil filled into her system and aviation spirit poured into her 75-gallon tanks.

With Segrave at the wheel, Willcocks and Halliwell hand-pumped water until it squirted from the vent cocks of the water-cooling system, closed cocks and returned to their seats either side of the pilot. Segrave switched on both engines and instructed his mechanics to press air-starter buttons and wind their hand magnetos. The engines went into action. Segrave signalled that the oil pressure was OK. The boat moved forwards. As speed increased, *Miss England II* lifted herself out of the water onto her step – 'climbing the hump' – and flattened out. Engine temperatures started to rise and the mechanics gradually opened the water discharge overboard, thus allowing water from the scoops to enter the water-cooling system. Three greasers above this were then operated to lubricate the top shafts of the engines, the gearbox and the inboard bearing of those top shafts. Each mechanic then held a card in his left hand with a pencil on a lanyard in his right hand and an attempt was made to take instrument readings.

Segrave decided to make this first run at only three-quarters throttle. With their helmets fitted with ear-pads and defenders inserted in their ears, the cockpit seemed virtually silent and everything had to be done by visual signals.

The first run had been fine and the boat slowed down to a mere 75mph for the turn. The pilot closed the throttles, put full helm to turn to starboard, and opened full throttle. *Miss*

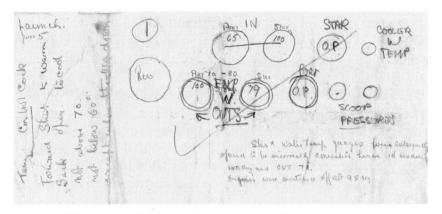

One of Willcocks' pencilled notes of the instruments. This, relating to control cocks, records that "the starboard water temperature gauges were subsequently found to be incorrectly connected, hence IN reading 100 deg and OUT 79. Engines were switched off at 95 deg". Each run was logged *(Michael Willcocks)*

*England II* banked to turn so fast that Willcocks' shoulder kept bumping the edge of the cockpit – which was made of special 'pneumatic' upholstery covered in red leather.

On the return run Willcocks recalled "There came a slight thud. I looked up at Sir Henry, who was sitting with both hands on the wheel. Yet both engines were switched off, spinning round, losing momentum. Both clutches were out. We were coasting to a standstill. Sir Henry said 'It's alright, I think we've broken something down aft. Prop shaft or something'."

"Vic Halliwell said, 'But you've got the clutches out!' and he and I were just goggling at each other in amazement. We were travelling at 107mph at the time of the breakage. The clutches, one for each engine, were operated by two levers, one on either side of Sir Henry's seat. He had to let go the wheel, holding it between his knees, operate two switches, lean forward, grasp the levers, depress two knobs on the top, pull them towards him past the hips and some inches behind him, release the knobs and put his two hands on the wheel again – all in the fraction of time it takes a normal person to lift his head!

"I looked at the wake trailing away behind us. It was as straight as a die. I have often thought back to my tasks in the cockpit of *Miss England II* and marvelled. You see, it was not merely physical action in that fraction of a second. The senses had to realise something was wrong, where it was, and the correct thing to do to prevent further damage, in a brand-new boat the second time out.

"It was hardly credible. One of the blades had broken off the two-bladed propeller while revolving at 12,000 rpm – 200 revs per second. But think of the speed of those messages to the brain and limb!"

*Miss England II* returned slowly to dock and her prop was taken off. On Tuesday evening at 7.45pm, another test was made with a new prop. After another good run south, a beautiful port turn and a return north at two-thirds throttle – they were nearing the American speed that they had to beat when they suddenly slowed off again. Another blade had snapped.

\* \* \*

Vic Halliwell, although very involved in his engines, still got time to play with his little son, while Michael Willcocks spent most of his spare time in 'Herberts', the local photograph and gramophone record shop. In the morning, a girl came into the shop to have a film developed. When asked for her name, she gave it as 'Miss P. England'. This was afterwards checked to be true.

On Wednesday evening, with the usual flotilla of spectator craft being told to move out of the way, with some being more obliging than others, *Miss England II* came out for her fourth run. A local reporter wrote of this run, "In the afterglow of the setting sun the boat showed up a greyish-blue against the white of its spray leaving a slight tremor on the water and hardly any wash – and the initial sound of the exhaust changed into little more than a loud purr."

Once again the double course. On the second run, they stopped again halfway to attend to a water-cooling defect, then continued at a low speed back to dock, where another examination took place. Confronted by a large group of pressmen, Segrave told them that they had only got two-thirds full power – but that a three-figure speed had been reached again.

The bronze-steel (or manganese bronze) alloy prop used for this last run was slightly thicker and softer than the ones in pure steel, with a diameter of 16 inches. It had been made hurriedly by F. Bamford & Co Ltd of Stockport and, although it had not snapped, its blades were pitted with tiny sand holes and the edges slightly bent. This still was not good enough. But on Thursday morning, on a preliminary trial, a blade of another

Stockport prop snapped off at a speed of less than 50mph. "Fred, this one couldn't even pull the skin off a rice pudding!" Segrave complained to his designer Cooper. A car was dispatched to Derby to collect a new steel prop of 65-ton tensile strength. It was an overnight journey, which showed the urgency of the situation.

So far, *Miss England II* just had not given her best to the thousands of spectators. With every trial something had gone wrong. Lord Wakefield was waiting for his pilot to break the record, not the props. The two timekeepers would have to leave in two days' time for the Isle of Man motor-cycle T.T. Races. The situation is best reported in a confidential letter, which Segrave sent to Lord Wakefield, dated 12th June 1930. It was typed on the Segraves' Kingston Hill letter-headed paper, but sent from 'The Old England Hotel' at Windermere:

Dear Lord Wakefield,

First of all many thanks indeed for your kind telegram.
Let me now give you the worst side of the picture first. We have been seriously held up by broken propellers for two days. These propellers were made to my own and Mr Cooper's specification and drawings, and when the first one had broken I sent it to the Rolls-Royce Company's metallurgist for chemical analysis, and we found that all the propellers made for me by Saunders-Roe, four in number, two of which have broken, and the other twisted, have been delivered to us by this firm 60% under strength, hence the breakage.

I have notified Saunders-Roe of this very serious matter which might have had disastrous consequences, because the blades instead of breaking off downwards from the hull might have gone through the bottom of the hull, sinking the boat immediately.

The Rolls-Royce Company are delivering a propeller tomorrow midday which we will fit at once and attempt a record in the afternoon at about 4pm.

"The propeller will not, however, enable the boat to attain its maximum speed because it will be too thick in the blade. I remember writing to you about six months ago in which letter I mentioned to you that I thought we should get the record back before the 15th June, and this promise I should like to adhere to.

If we are successful tomorrow I propose to leave the Boat here and return to London whilst the English Steel Corporation make us an ultra high tensile steel propeller which will take about 14 days. Then we would return here and bring the timekeepers up here again and show the real speed of which the boat is capable.

At the present moment, on rather less then two-thirds of the full power I have been over a 100mph, and the record stands at 92.86mph. The boat trims and handles absolutely perfectly and is in every way a complete success, our only trouble being the propeller.

I will wire you tomorrow and let you know what happens.

Yours sincerely,

H.O.D. Segrave.

That evening, a typewritten notice was issued to each member of the team. It read: "*Miss England II* will attempt the record tomorrow afternoon at 4pm. She will run between the pylons on the west or Lancashire shore of the lake and within one hundred yards of the buoys."

"This boat can murder the record," Segrave told a reporter. "The only difficulty is that we have not yet found a propeller that will stand up to full power ... I have kept people waiting a long time. There are thousands of people interested and I feel I have got to go out and put up a show tomorrow."

# 8

# Friday, 13<sup>th</sup> June 1930

When Segrave half strolled, half limped down the jetty to feed a swan on the morning of Friday 13<sup>th</sup> of June, the sun was already shining and the crowds had begun to gather on the banks of Windermere. A reporter approached him to ask him about the dangers of the project he was undertaking. He replied that if, during an attempt, they were to be thrown out of the boat, the water would be as hard as a board. In fact, they had even taken precautions against this danger. Special armoured lifejackets, consisting of flexible strips of steel enclosed in material had been ordered from Guires of Cowes, but as yet only one had arrived. Segrave refused to have an unfair advantage over his mechanics. If they could not wear them, then he certainly would not.

"I am nervous about today's attempt," Lady Doris Segrave explained. "I feel that something may happen. I don't know how to explain it but there is something that tells me that things are amiss ... Again and again he has touched wood, but one cannot go on tempting fate."

By midday, thousands of people were massed around the course on Windermere, many lining the promenade at Bowness, others by the shore, on the islands and on the various craft that were floating offshore. Hundreds had pairs of binoculars hanging around their necks. The sun was shining gloriously. Segrave, in immaculate overalls, was offered one of the St Bartholemew Hospital car mascots to attach to his boat. He refused it with the comment, "I would not have a mascot at any price."

He talked to reporters: "Well, now for it! She has chewed up some propellers, and I am trying a bronze one on her now. If this fails I shall put a steel one on, and if that fails I shall postpone my attempt for a week or so to make experiments with a new prop. The boat is an absolute experiment and anything may happen but we have got to trust to luck and the wonderful skill of those who have been working on her for so long."

Lifejackets were fixed and helmets put on. As he was about to climb onto the boat, Segrave is reported to have patted an old friend, the journalist Harold Pemberton, on the back and remarked, "Pem, old lad, I'm going to do it this time. I'm not going to let anyone down again."

At 1.15pm, *Miss England II* was towed out from her wet dock by *Miss London* to save any stress on her new propeller: a bronze one. Michael Willcocks was to recall, "On the way out, Sir Henry made an alteration in the programme. Instead of returning to the boathouse after a run in each direction to fit the other propeller, he decided to do two runs at only just over record speed. 'You and I, Halliwell,' he said to Vic, 'will take the times of the first run, and if not good enough for the average, I will increase slightly on the return. Then if everything is OK, I'll run her up again all out, and see how much over 120 she'll do. I hope to Heaven she'll behave herself.'

"I said, 'She'll be alright, sir. Friday the 13th is my lucky day.' Sir Henry smiled and said 'That's something anyway'."

Willcocks was not to know that fifteen years before, during the First World War, Second Lieutenant H.O.D. Segrave had been ordered to occupy a captured trench with sixty men during the Battle of Neuve-Chapelle – and got there with fourteen. The date was 'The close of the 13th, one of the unluckiest days I have ever lived through.'

As one of the 'Lost Generation', Segrave had survived. He had also survived the dangers of record-breaking where fellow competitors like the Welshman Parry Thomas and the American Lee Bible had suffered fatal injuries trying to break the records he had set up. It was perhaps only natural that he was known to have made such statements as, "I have one chance in ten. But I have become a fatalist. I take all possible precautions. After that I become a fatalist. If everything is right, I try. If I win, I win – if I fail, I fail."

And of the *Miss England II* venture, he is supposed to have described it as, "The greatest gamble of my life. Call it a gamble with death if you like."

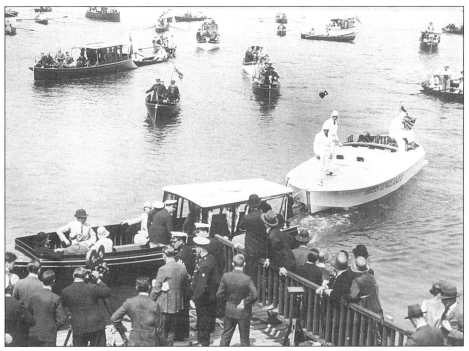

Always exposed to full public and media glare *(Author's collection)*

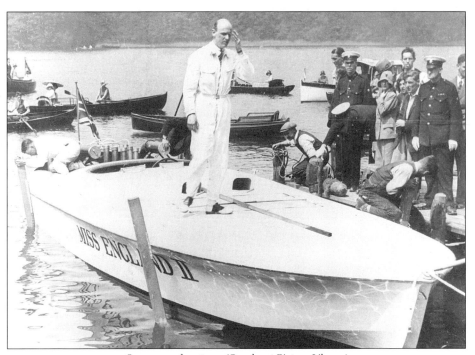

Segrave under stress *(Quadrant Picture Library)*

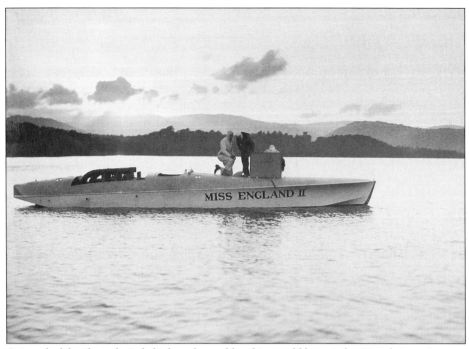

Out on the lake, the technical glitches of record-breaking could be sorted out in relative privacy ... *(Michael Willcocks)*

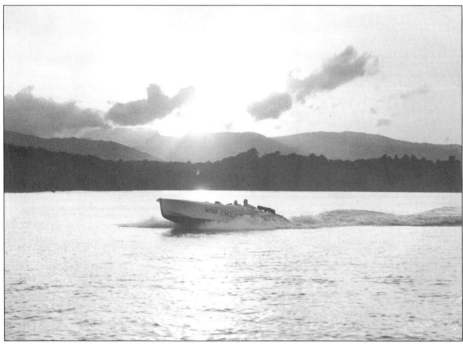

... for the crew to come back to dock at the end of a fine day's work *(Author's collection)*

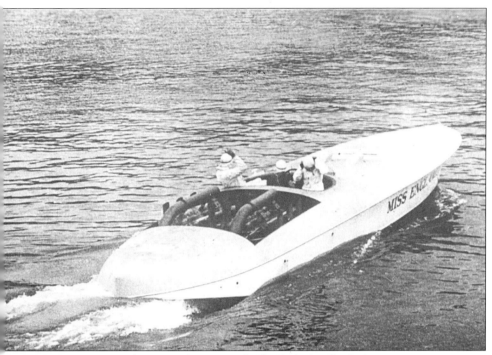

Heading out to the Measured Mile *(Author's collection)*

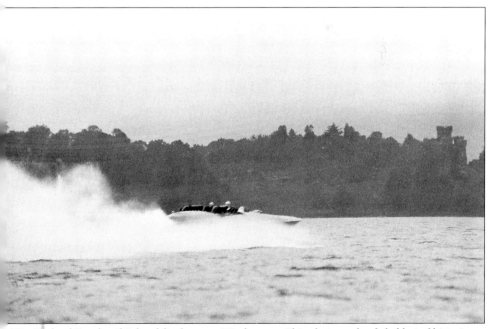

*Miss England II* on her third and final run on Windermere. This photograph – faded but of historic importance – was taken only seconds before the crash. The gothic silhouette of Wray Castle on Windermere's western shore adds to the atmosphere *(Michael Willcocks)*

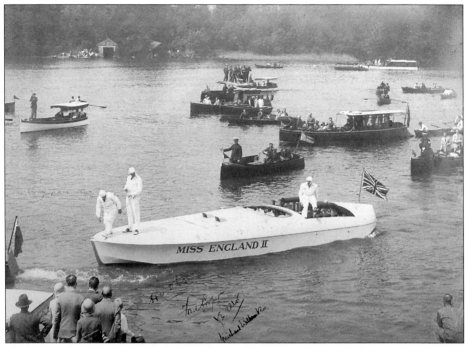

Photograph of *Miss England II*, autographed by the team on Thursday 12th June, prior to the accident *(Windermere Motor Boat Racing Club)*

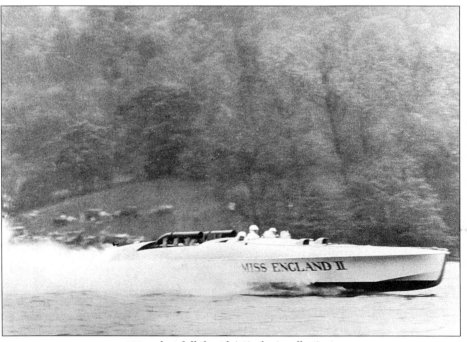

120 mph at full throttle! *(Author's collection)*

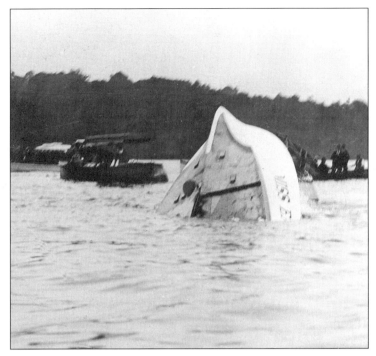

Bows up and going
down
*(Author's
collection)*

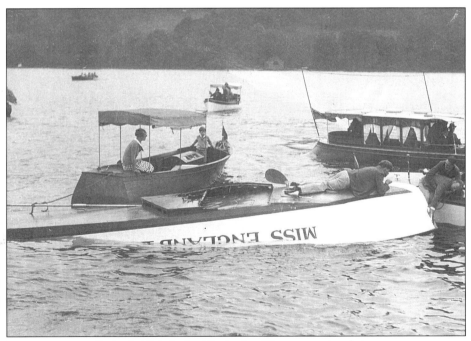

Trying to hitch the boat for towing. Observe punctured step
*(Allied Newspapers – author's collection)*

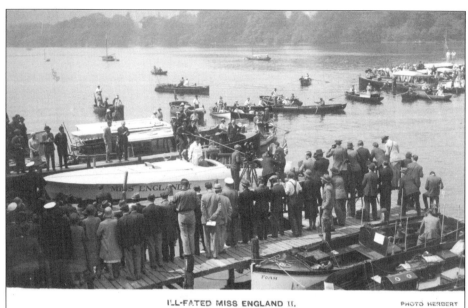

ILL-FATED MISS ENGLAND II.

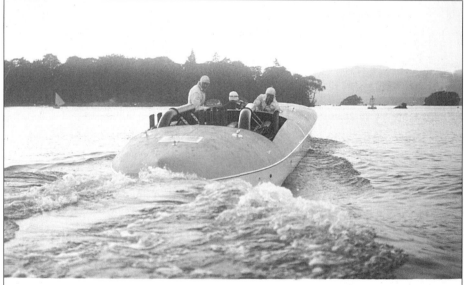

ILL FATED MISS ENGLAND II. ON WINDERMERE.

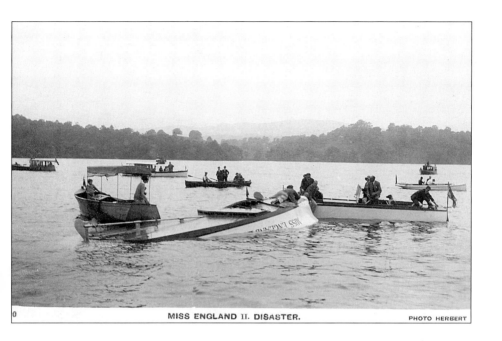

MISS ENGLAND II. DISASTER. PHOTO HERBERT

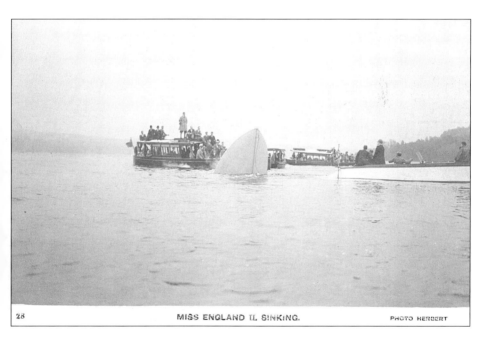

MISS ENGLAND II. SINKING. PHOTO HERBERT

Herbert & Sons, Photographers of Windermere, had a superb sequence of shots, which as postcards, sold very well. Those shown on these two pages succeed in capturing the sequence of events on 13th June.

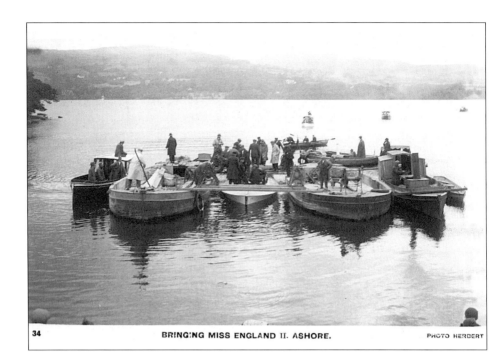

34        BRINGING MISS ENGLAND II. ASHORE.        PHOTO HERBERT

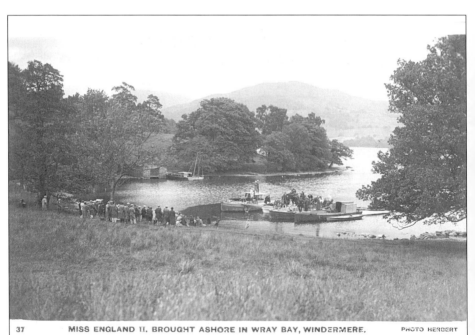

37      MISS ENGLAND II. BROUGHT ASHORE IN WRAY BAY, WINDERMERE.      PHOTO HERBERT

Two further postcards from the Herbert & Sons' collection

*Miss England II* cast off. Starting procedure was begun. All binoculars and movie cameras were trained onto the accelerating boat. The timekeepers were poised. The Police and Club launches were attempting to keep back the flotilla. "We were keyed up and tense," Willcocks recalled. "We knew that anything might happen but we were taking the risk."

She shot across the Mile. Turned and returned at a faster speed against the wind, but riding the water almost dead flat. Crossing the southerly marker buoy, she overran the finishing point by nearly a mile, Segrave pointed to his stopwatch with both thumbs up. Not only had the prop held, but they'd almost definitely broken the record. So with a spectacular starboard turn, 'showing two rainbows of spray ... and the humming of her engines echoing and re-echoing among the hills,' the white speedboat took a half-a-mile run-up and shot across the buoy again. Segrave literally stood on the throttle pedals.

"There was a glorious feeling of 'kissing' the surface at slightly less than one second intervals with the timely little flick of the stern, fore and aft and sideways – a grand feeling," said Willcocks. "One has a similar feeling in a plane just as the wings are taking the full weight of the machine. I glanced at Sir Henry, smiling and very obviously delighted. As we ran for the line, I grinned and flicked a few fingers to Joe Chamberlain of the Wakefield Oil Company."

*Miss England II* was travelling extremely fast when, reaching the middle of the course, she struck something. In Willcocks' words, "Then there was a slight thud from for'ard, a slight list and swerve to port. We straightened, then to starboard again, and straightened again. The bows were rising up ... she oughtn't do this ... going over, water coming up to meet ... Bang!"

According to press reports, "Suddenly there was a bump – the boat swerved to port. A grim look came into Segrave's face and his body became taut as he pulled at the wheel to correct, or overcorrect, for the boat then swerved to starboard in a cloud of spray. There was a moment and her engines were silenced as she turned turtle.

"The boat turned over clockwise – Halliwell on the port side got the strongest throw and was seen flying in a great arc. Segrave was in the centre of it – Willcocks was only tipped into the water. There was that terrible swerve and she seemed to drive like a bullet beneath the waters."

The complete and shocked silence was broken by the shrill laughter that came from someone in a pleasure launch who could not have seen the tragedy. Waking from their state of shock, several boats at once converged on the upturned craft and its crew. Halliwell was already sinking when the first one arrived. Willcocks was 'doggy-paddling' in panic to keep himself up.

Philip King, of nearby Troutbeck, caught sight of a bald head occasionally submerged beneath the waves of the approaching craft, his hands waving feebly. Diving in, fully clothed, he grabbed Segrave by his clothing and pulled him back to his launch. He was taken to Belle Grange, a private house on the Lancashire side of the lake, where Lady Doris, who had watched the trials from the shore, rushed to his side. Both his arms and two ribs were broken, one thigh badly crushed, his head injured and one eye out. Though in great pain he was still conscious and had already asked after his mechanics' safety. He asked his wife if he had got the record and received a grief-stricken affirmative. It hurts terribly to speak with badly broken ribs, but Segrave then asked by how much he had beaten it. Although it took time to find the official timekeepers, eventually the figure was brought back to him. When told the new record of 98.76mph, Segrave – according to one Italian magazine – is reported to have remarked, "Ora si po pure morire" = "Now one can die."

The three doctors at his side could not do anything. Sir Henry Segrave died at 5 o'clock, after three hours of consciousness and pain. One of the broken ribs had punctured his lung, causing a haemorrhage. He was 34 years old.

Percy Duff was eight years old at the time: "We didn't see the crash as it happened further up the lake, but I remember a boat coming back to Bowness and the great cheer when Willcocks raised his hand to show us he was alright."

Meanwhile, all that was left of *Miss England II* was a wide patch of oil and hundreds of ping-pong balls which had escaped from her buoyancy bags. When the rescue or press launches had approached, she had been upturned. Someone tried to attach a rope to her bows so they could tow her to the shore. But in the effort, water had flooded into her aft. With that, and the weight of the engines, soon all that remained of her above water was her bows – pointing vertically upwards. She sank completely after only fifteen minutes.

They had to give up looking for Halliwell at midnight. But after another two days' search, they picked up his body. He was still wearing his goggles and still clutching the pencil and paper on which were notes of the engine's revs on that last run. These notes confirmed that *Miss England II* had attained an unofficial 119.8mph on that final burst of speed. This made her the fastest boat in the world.

Willcocks, black and blue, with a damaged spine, a massive bruise on his thigh and a knee-to-ankle gash on his left leg, was soon nursed back to health and went on to help with salvage operations. Even today, the many loose pieces of driftwood on the pebble shore suggest the possible cause of the accident – 'possible' because, even after almost 70 years, several contradictory rumours circulate around Windermere as to what gave way to what. As has already been mentioned, the front step was adjustable; althoughit was separate from the hull proper, it was fixed on with over eighty specially made stainless steel nuts and bolts, but it was possible to correct the trim of the boat by a fractional alteration.

Since the accident, there have been lingering question marks about this adjustability: had one of the bolts snapped off just before the attempt and, rather than unscrew all the others, had they cut out a surrounding piece and bolted in a makeshift one? Hadn't the bolts been tightened up before the attempt – as in all previous trials? Another idea that was formulated at the time by a 'lay' journalist was that the gearbox had burst! But such an event would have immediately sunk the boat.

During the rest of that afternoon, whilst the weather was turning contrastingly gloomy, two pieces of evidence were found which were to contribute to the likely cause of the accident. Firstly, there was a waterlogged branch measuring about 3 feet long and 3 inches thick with three fresh 'grazes' or marks. This had apparently been found, twenty minutes after the crash (when most of the flotilla had dispersed) about 250 yards behind what could be estimated as the third path of the boat. Secondly, a couple of hours later, part of the missing step, shaped like an axe, which had also been floating but weighted under water, was brought back to land.

When, after a fortnight, they had located the boat, and – after trial and error – had found the right equipment for lifting her, it took them two days to tow her back to shore. A full inspection was made. The log seemed to fit with the axe-shaped part of the step, which in turn seemed to fit the rest of the step. In the inquest which followed, the verdict was 'Accidental Death.'

Willcocks recalled that, "It was not a very large room and it was full to capacity. Very few Press were there as far as I know. The Coroner was very decent to me and I was able to say exactly what happened, in my own words. There were various views about which way the boat turned over. I said 'Well, the boat turned over to starboard, I was on the starboard side.'"

The best explanation of what may have actually happened has been given by the well-known naval architect Uffa Fox in his book 'Sail and Power':

"It was towards the end of this run that she most unfortunately struck a submerged log, which pierced a hole in her forward step ... the water at 120 miles an hour pressure rushed into this hole and set up an enormous water pressure inside the port step. Planing along at 120mph, *Miss England II* was only riding on the after end of this step, and the after end of the aft step. The water pressure from without was thus only taking place on the aft end of her steps, so that the water had entered and was still entering the hole with great force and it could not force off the after end of the step; but it could and did rush into the forepart, and there, with nothing to resist its outward pressure, it in effect blew the forepart of the port side downwards and outwards, till finally that forepart was torn completely off. The capsizing moment of this part of the step as it was being torn downwards and off, was sufficient, as can easily be imagined, to roll *Miss England* right over."

Also to this day, people are still not sure who had made the final, unbreakable, record-breaking propeller. Saunders-Roe? Rolls-Royce? Bamfords of Stockport? Each company would make the claim.

Segrave had once declared, "Speed will be the keynote of the world in the future and this country has got to lead if it is going to live. Nor does speed always mean speed for speed's sake. It means, as any engineer appreciates, the discovery of all those factors that make better engines, more power for less weight, improved springing, cleaner body design, and all the 101 points which make mechanical developments possible. So when an accident happens, it is no use saying, 'What's the use?' There is a use. It is towards someone, something and the less known may be worth all the risks and losses.

"If I go out, may it be doing something worthwhile. I do not want to die between the sheets. I would go out with my boots on!"

The following message was sent to Lady Segrave by Lord Stamfordhalm on behalf of King George and Queen Mary:

> It is with much regret that the King and Queen have learned of the tragic death of Sir Henry Segrave. I am commanded to convey to you the expression of their Majesties' heartfelt sympathy in your irreparable loss. The King recalls with pleasure the occasion at Bognor Regis when he conferred a knighthood on Sir Henry, and his Majesty mourns the death of one whose intrepid adventures on land and water were the admiration of all the world.

It as a tragedy noted in many a diary. Among those living in the Lake District at the time was a 46-year-old foreign news correspondent by name of Arthur Ransome. Ransome was working on the manuscript of a children's novel which, with the title of 'Swallows and Amazons' would earn him an enduring world fame. His diary entry for June 13<sup>th</sup> reads:

> Molly went back. Returning from the station after seeing her off learned that Segrave's boat sunk with one of his engineers, Segrave and the other engineer rescued badly injured.

This was followed by the June 14<sup>th</sup> entry:

> Segrave died from his injuries two hours after the accident.

The funeral took place at Golders Green Crematorium in north-west London. It was a very private affair. Only the closest friends of the family were present. Elsewhere, on the same day, there was a more public memorial service at St Margaret's, Westminster. Later that year, Segrave's ashes were taken up in the Segrave Meteor monoplane by his father and, at Lady Segrave's request, scattered over the playing fields of Eton

Public School, where he had spent some of the happiest years of his life.

After salvage, the rest of *Miss England II*'s hull was taken down to Rolls-Royce in Derby to be thoroughly cleaned out, dried out, and examined. The only renewals needed were the step and where the grappling wires of the salvage boats had chafed – and in some places – broken the light hatches and coamings on the deck. The engines had already been stripped and cleaned and they were reinstalled.

Soon, people began to wonder whether Segrave's hydro-plane was bound for some museum or whether Lord Wakefield would let a new pilot continue her achievements. Wakefield was so upset by the death of Sir Henry Segrave, whom he had virtually regarded as his own son, that for a time it looked as if *Miss England II* would be joining her sister ship *Miss England I*, now on view in the Science Museum in London, as a gift to the nation.

# 9

# Kaye Don

If the *Miss England II* project were to continue, several choices would have to be made. Who would replace Segrave? Who would replace Halliwell? Where would she run? A potential pilot was Count Johnston-Noad, a 30-year-old millionaire who had won the Duke of York's 1½ litre Gold Motorboat Trophy in 1924 and 1928; he announced his intention to build a Saunders-Napier hydroplane, *Miss Empire III*, and to break Segrave's record on Gairloch in Scotland. The attempt was part of Count Noad's plan to win the Triple Crown and so become the fastest man on land, air and water within the same year. Castrol were on the point of backing him when Lord Wakefield changed his mind.

The alternative pilot recommended to Lord Wakefield was a successful racing driver called Kaye Don. In many ways, the career of Kaye Ernest Don (shortened from the Polish Donsky) was very similar to Segrave's, except that whereas Segrave's luck had held until the end, Don had always seemed to be dogged by bad luck. He was born in Dublin on 1st April 1891 and educated at Wolverhampton Grammar School. His father died when he was only 17, and Don had to forsake University and take a position as a junior clerk in the offices of a tyre company, with a mother and a sister entirely dependant on him. He still found time, however, to compete in many reliability trials with motorcycles.

Although he joined the Army in 1915, he was discharged nine months later on medical grounds. Like Segrave, Don then learned to fly and served as a Lieutenant (RFC) on the Western Front. In March 1919, he was transferred to Ireland for light duty. He took out his own motorcycle and sidecar and, with an observer, was engaged in various minor detail work.

After the armistice, he entered motorcycle racing and made the fastest speed of 71mph at Kop Hill, England and in 1920 did five miles at an average of 69.82mph. Both these speeds were considered very fast at the time. Motorcycling began to lose interest for Don and he took up motor racing at Brooklands Track and on the Continent. He began racing a light A.C. 4-cylinder car, breaking the hour record at over 90mph in 1922. During the years that followed, he became very busy as sales manager of his tyre company, but continued racing round the Brooklands banking at speeds approaching 130mph. In 1928, for example, driving a 2-litre red Sunbeam, Don won the President's Gold Plate and the Gold Star at 118mph for 25 miles. He did not drive spectacularly – just cornering at hair-raising speeds, passing other cars with 2 inches to spare, and double-skidding round corners. He became one of the idols of Brooklands. Don also won the RAC International Tourist Trophy at Ulster at an average speed of 64mph. This race was one of the most thrilling runs of his career for, in a 410-mile drive, he won by only 13 seconds.

Don's experience on the water began in the April of 1929, when he attempted to set up a national speed record for unlimited outboard motorboats. Piloting a 10ft bob-sled-shaped hull, powered by a supercharged Dunelt engine, he was clocked at 22.5mph – unfortunately not enough for a new outboard record. A couple of months later, Don planned to make the double crossing between Dover and Calais in under one hour. The Royal Speedboat Company at Poole gave him one of their 30ft standard models, powered by a 200hp Kermath engine, which he called the 'Kaye Don Special'. On Tuesday 23rd July at 3.30 in the morning and against the advice of local fishermen, Don and his three-man crew moved out over a very stormy Channel and into a south-westerly gale. About two miles out and at a speed of 45mph, they hit a huge wave. With a shattered windscreen and faltering engine, the crippled craft limped back to Dover Harbour. Three days later, with the boat repaired and in calmer weather, they completed the double trip in 1 hour 23 minutes, lowering the 1927 record by 24 minutes.

That same year, after winning almost every major class record for racing cars, including a new kilometre record for Brooklands of 140.95mph, Kaye Don decided to go for the World Unlimited Land Speed Record. In January 1930, the

4,000hp Sunbeam-engined Silver Bullet car, designed by Louis Coätelen was taken to Pendine Sands, where it could only reach a top speed of 158mph. In March, Don was only able to improve that figure to an official two-way average of 183mph on Daytona Beach, Florida – not enough to beat the existing 231mph record. He returned to Ireland to drive an Alfa-Romeo in the gruelling 410-mile Ulster T.T. race and was cornering superbly when he skidded at 70mph and was crushed beneath his overturned car. He was badly bruised and burnt, eight ribs fractured and a smashed shoulder blade, with his back and sides badly lacerated. He was unable to drive for the rest of the 1930 season.

In November of that year, 'Lonny' Limb, the racing manager at Castrol and a good friend of Kaye Don, suggested the tall, 39-year-old speed merchant to Lord Wakefield as Segrave's logical successor. By December 1930 the venture was again underway with a projected attack on the record in a regatta which the Argentine Yacht Club was to hold during the British Empire Exhibition at Buenos Aires in the spring of 1931.

*Miss England II* had been miraculously located and recovered from a depth of 180ft without the use of divers. They succeeded in ingeniously slinging four steel-wire ropes between two barges and under the hull of the boat, and winching her to the surface. Filled with mud and debris, the soiled speedboat was taken down to Derby for a thorough overhaul and modifications. This time there must be no accidents. Her hull bottom was to be sheathed in $\frac{1}{16}$-inch stainless steel to avoid the initial penetration of her step, which started the Windermere crash. The throttle controls were interconnected so that control was through a single accelerator pedal.

*Miss England II* was re-fitted in a Rolls-Royce engineering workshop next to a bay where two employees had spent twenty years making sure that the bonnets of Rolls-Royce cars fitted perfectly – and nothing else. Willcocks recalled: "They'd lift the bonnet up and if it wasn't quite right, they'd file it until it closed down flush. It would have driven me up the wall. Cracking stones on Dartmoor was preferable to that!"

Once ready, there was a Press Day. The re-conditioned speedboat with its original engines 'running even better than ever', to use an official description, was photographed over a hundred times and pictures were taken of the roaring engines. Willcocks spoke into the microphone, "We are carrying on where we left off.

"I described the installation and the cockpit. Then, they made me do it again. I pity the actresses who have to say the same thing over and over again in the movie studios."

Alonso Limb of Castrol declared, "This is a triumph for the

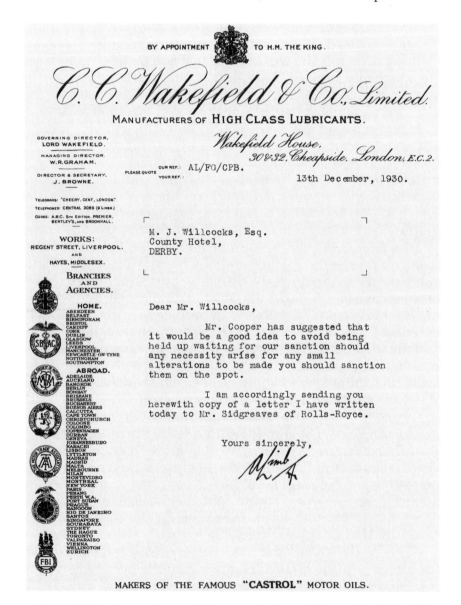

BY APPOINTMENT TO H.M. THE KING.

## C. C. Wakefield & Co., Limited.

### MANUFACTURERS OF HIGH CLASS LUBRICANTS.

GOVERNING DIRECTOR.
**LORD WAKEFIELD.**

MANAGING DIRECTOR.
**W. R. GRAHAM.**

DIRECTOR & SECRETARY,
**J. BROWNE.**

*Wakefield House,*
*30 & 32, Cheapside, London, E.C.2.*

PLEASE QUOTE OUR REF.: AL/FG/CPB.
YOUR REF.:

13th December, 1930.

TELEGRAMS: "CHEERY, CENT, LONDON."
TELEPHONES: CENTRAL 3089 (9 LINES.)
CODES: A.B.C. 5TH EDITION, PREMIER, BENTLEY'S, AND BROOMHALL.

**WORKS:**
REGENT STREET, LIVERPOOL.
AND
HAYES, MIDDLESEX.

**BRANCHES**
AND
**AGENCIES.**

**HOME.**
ABERDEEN
BELFAST
BIRMINGHAM
BRISTOL
CARDIFF
CORK
DUBLIN
GLASGOW
LEEDS
LIVERPOOL
MANCHESTER
NEWCASTLE-ON-TYNE
NOTTINGHAM
SOUTHAMPTON

**ABROAD.**
ADELAIDE
AUCKLAND
BANGKOK
BERLIN
BOMBAY
BRISBANE
BRUSSELS
BUCHAREST
BUENOS AIRES
CALCUTTA
CAPE TOWN
CHRISTCHURCH
COLOGNE
COLOMBO
COPENHAGEN
DURBAN
GENEVA
JOHANNESBURG
KARACHI
LISBON
LYTTLETON
MADRAS
MADRID
MALTA
MELBOURNE
MILAN
MONTEVIDEO
MONTREAL
NEW YORK
PARIS
PENANG
PERTH W.A.
PORT SUDAN
PRAGUE
RANGOON
RIO DE JANEIRO
SANTOS
SINGAPORE
SOURABAYA
SYDNEY
THE HAGUE
TORONTO
VALPARAISO
VIENNA
WELLINGTON
ZURICH

M. J. Willcocks, Esq.
County Hotel,
DERBY.

Dear Mr. Willcocks,

Mr. Cooper has suggested that it would be a good idea to avoid being held up waiting for our sanction should any necessity arise for any small alterations to be made you should sanction them on the spot.

I am accordingly sending you herewith copy of a letter I have written today to Mr. Sidgreaves of Rolls-Royce.

Yours sincerely,

*Limb*

**MAKERS OF THE FAMOUS "CASTROL" MOTOR OILS.**

Michael Willcocks was given permission to authorise small jobs on *Miss England II*, following a request to Rolls-Royce. This letter from Alonso Limb confirmed the arrangement *(Michael Willcocks)*

Rolls-Royce works, done well within the scheduled time by a small army of men who have been engaged on the task. As the second riding mechanic we have decided to choose Mr Richard Garner of Rolls-Royce.

"Mr Garner, who is 21 years old, is the son of Mr Charles Garner, canvasser and collector for the Midland Railway at Derby. Richard Garner has lived at Darley Dale in Nottingham, where he attended the High Pavement School. By dint of hard work and study, he secured scholarships and at the age of fifteen commenced his apprenticeship at the Rolls-Royce works in Derby. Mr Garner has shown exceptional merit in his work, and his capabilities have been recognised by the distinction now accorded him. He is an all-round sportsman, being connected with the Derby Rowing Club and the Rolls-Royce Hockey team. Everyone will wish him the best of luck and success in his connection with the attempt on the speed record." Willcocks' only concern was that Garner was so young.

Although Kaye Don had begun to get in some high-speed hydroplaning on the Solent in a 60mph craft called *Crescendo*, it was obvious that some freshwater course would have to be found where he could get the particular feel of *Miss England II* at speed. Michael Willcocks, who had bravely decided to get back in a boat that had almost killed him, was asked to reconnoitre a location near Derby. He had rejected a nearby reservoir as unsuitable because it was surrounded by baulks of loose timber, when Castrol decided to ship *Miss England II* out to Lough Neagh, near Belfast, Northern Ireland. Willcocks went out with an advanced guard and selected a clear course on the north-east part of the water, near the South Antrim golf links.

Shipped over on the *Ulster Queen*, *Miss England II* was put on a solid-tyred steam wagon which took her to the lough at a speed of just under 3mph – the slowest speed she'd ever done. Willcocks recalled: "I couldn't stand that. It was too slow. So they loaned me an Austin Twelve and I went on ahead."

This time, experts, mechanics, hydrographers and aeroplane pilots were sent over to inspect the Lough. A large steam dredger scraped the entire length of the course. Nets were dragged over the shallower water whilst an aeroplane flew overhead, scanning the depths for any water-logged, semi-submerged objects.

Although the programme of one month's working-up trials had been planned, Don, with Willcocks and Garner as his racing mechanics, was dogged by bad weather. The dampness played havoc with the sparking plugs of the Rolls-Royce engines. On January 20th the drizzle lifted. Don had gone off to play golf. A telephone call was made from the boathouse to the golf course and a caddy rushed over the links. Don dropped his clubs, motored back to the lake-side and was in the boat within a quarter of an hour. He drove *Miss England II* in figures-of-eight at around 40mph. Two days later, at dusk, he was also able to make a couple of 80mph sprints. As one journalist wrote: "Indeed, his mastery of the boat after not more than 20 minutes aboard was most impressive. The preliminary tests have proved so satisfactory that Don intends to make a high-speed trial today, his objective being 115mph."

But from then on, a raging gale prevented further runs, the Press decided to go home and, on January 24th, the trials were abandoned. Of these aborted trials, Willcocks would later recall: "When I was in Ireland, I tore a strip off a member of the team who should have known better than to say anything in any shape or form to the disparagement of Segrave. I told him off properly in front of a lot of people. I was being paid not to say those sort of things. The Castrol Manager, Alonso Limb, said, 'You did not behave very well in Ireland.'

"I thought I did my job correctly."

"Well Don drives a car around Brooklands that nobody else will drive. He's a very good man."

"I don't know anything about him. I'm seeing this job through to the end because Segrave would have wished it."

"There are hundreds of people who would jump at your job."

"Get one. I don't mind in the least."

*Miss England II* had only just been sent back to England, when it became known she was to be shipped to the Argentine, where, at Buenos Aires, Don was to drive her over a 10-mile course and make a new attempt on the Record.

# 10

# Argentina

During the 1920s Argentina was the only advanced country in Latin America. But in 1930, the Republic had undergone a political revolution. In September of that year, police had fired into a crowd of demonstrating law and medical students from the University of Buenos Aires and killed one of them. On September 6th the Argentinean people woke to the drone of military aircraft and knew that a revolution was on. The radical long-term President, Hipolito Yrigoyen, was overthrown and, from the 8th September, replaced by a military provisional government under General José Felix Uriburu.

Under this regime, Great Britain and the USA began to compete for the Argentinean market. For this reason, the British had organised an 'Exposicion Britanica', a British Empire Trade Exhibition at Buenos Aires where, with HRH Edward the Prince of Wales as patron, every British manufactured product from a pin to a locomotive was on display.

With Lord Wakefield's continued sponsorship, Don's mission was to bring *Miss England II* to the Argentine and by demonstrating a high-performance British hydroplane in action, so boost prestige from the water. Whilst the Speed King left London for Buenos Aires in February 1931 on the *Andalucia Star*, his crew and *Miss England II* took ship on board the *Stuart Star*, a ship regularly transporting beef from South America, but with a capacity for fifteen passengers.

Willcocks recalled: "On the way out, they were using coal stored in the several meat holds. As soon as each hold was emptied, they would wash it down thoroughly, paint everything, sterilise the hooks and put the refrigerator to work." *Miss England II* was lashed down to the deck and protected with canvas covers marked 'Lord Wakefield of Hythe', on both port

```
Form No. 31.
   Blue Star Line (1920) Limited.
                                          No. on Passenger List _____ 4
   " S.S. Stuart Star "                   No. en la lista de Pasajeros _____

              ARGENTINE IMMIGRATION ORDER.
        ORDEN DE INMIGRACIÓN ARGENTINO.

   Name of Passenger    Mr. Michael Willcocks
   Nombre del Pasajero

   and                              Members of Family.
   y                               Miembros de su Familia.
```

Willcocks' immigration ticket on the *Stuart Star* liner *(Michael Willcocks)*

and starboard sides. Owing to heavy seas and resultant rolling of the ship, it was only possible on three occasions to examine and turn the two Rolls-Royce engines. Instead the team amused themselves by playing deck tennis, pontoon and poker on the three-week transatlantic voyage.

Arrangements had been made at Buenos Aires for *Miss England II* to be launched off the *Stuart Star* into the Rio de la Plata (the River Plate) and towed up to Tigre, an up-river holiday resort about 12 miles north-west of Buenos Aires. The river becomes the River Parana which, at 3,900 km (2,440 miles) is the second longest river in South America, As the hydroplane had been dispatched without propshaft and prop being fitted, she had to be temporarily stored on a barge called the *Argentino* where those essential components were fitted. The following day, the *Stuart Star*'s derrick lifted *Miss England II* on a cradle and lowered her into the river without any mishap.

Kaye Don, Willcocks and Garner started off up-river. Willcocks recalled, "We were towed through the filth of the Buenos Aires harbour. Then, after two hours, a strong wind blew up and it was hard going up the Parana until it became too rough to go any further. We'd have foundered if she had continued. The *Argentino* was advised to go into the same base where the *Eagle* aircraft carrier was. As we went in under her counter, they recognised the hydroplane. They were shouting 'Segrave! Segrave!'. Kaye Don was sitting in the cockpit at the time. I'd been in the Navy and I knew that you always stood to attention. So I got Garner and myself up upon the foredeck, and we stood to attention."

Unknown as yet to the *Miss England II* team, that very day, March 20ᵗʰ, Commodore Gar Wood had taken *Miss America IX*, her Packard engines now supercharged to develop a total 2,800 horsepower, out onto his private 'test track', along the Indian River, Florida, and set up a new three-way average of 102.25mph, thus becoming the first man in the world to average 100mph in a boat. Segrave's fatal record no longer stood. Don's reaction was 'That's fine! Now we've got something to go for.'

That night, *Miss England II* was moored at the Yacht Club Argentino. Willcocks had to sleep on board, in case the speed-boat was leaking. The following morning she finally arrived at Tigre, known to the resident British population as 'the Argentine Henley'. She was moored on the Rio Lujan at the landing stage of the Corporación Tiluca, local agents for America's leading mahogany sports boat manufacturer, the Chris-Craft Corporation.

The team booked into the Tigre Hotel, next door to the casino and on the other side of the river to the Chris-Craft boathouse. That weekend, *Miss England II* was prepared for her first run and her engines given a satisfactory trial of two minutes. All arrangements had been made for the runs to take place on the Rio Parana de Las Palmas at a course surveyed and equipped with electrically synchronised timing apparatus by the Argentinean Navy in association with the Yacht Club Argentino. As this official course was approximately 18 miles from Tigre, this was to require a tow of at least three hours up a delta cutting every time a high-speed run was attempted.

For miles, the Parana's banks were fringed by dense South American jungle. Rotten trees and logs were constantly falling into its current, forming treacherous islands of weed and driftwood and making *Miss England II*'s runway more like a floating obstacle course. Willcocks recalled, "I'll always remember grabbing at a branch that was going past the boat and finding the other end had got a tree on it! These hazards were not at all pleasant, but as other motorboats with scoops behaved satisfactorily, we decided to tow up to Parana for a first high-speed run. On the Parana, the Argentine Navy had placed their gunboat

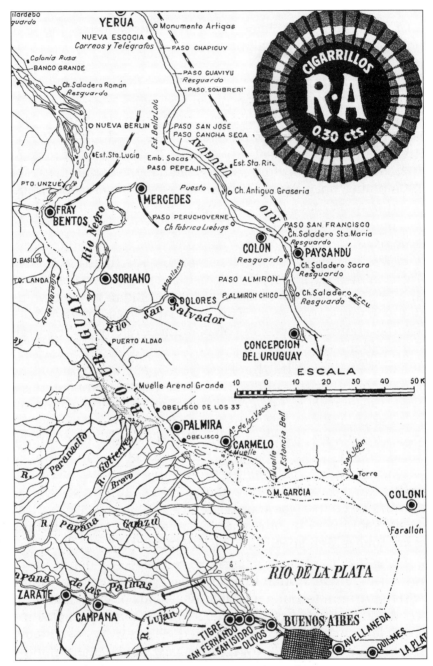

A 1930 map of the rivers Paraná and Uruguay and their tributaries. The funnel-shaped bay of the River Plate (Rio de la Plata) leads to one of the several arms of the River Paraná. Observant readers will note the hand-drawn line alongside the river (between Campana and the estuary leading into the bay) that was drawn by Willcocks to denote the course *(Michael Willcocks)*

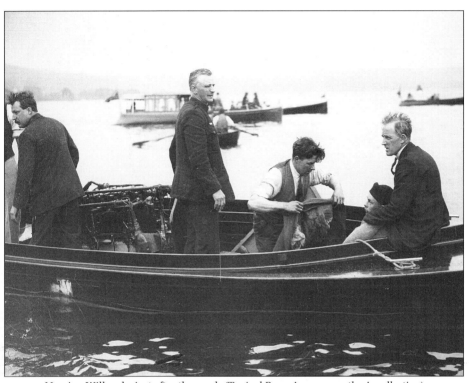

Nursing Willcocks just after the crash *(Topical Press Agency – author's collection)*

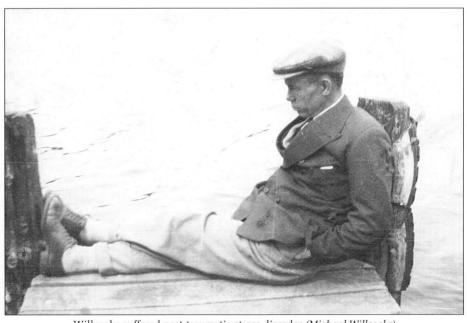

Willcocks suffered post-traumatic stress disorder *(Michael Willcocks)*

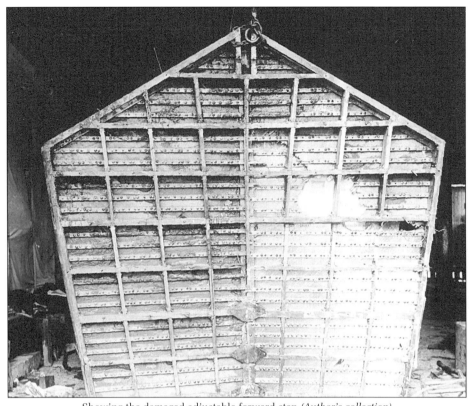

Showing the damaged adjustable forward step *(Author's collection)*

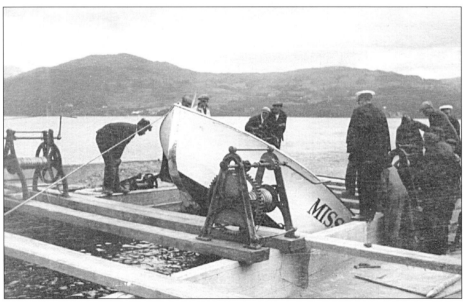

Raising the boat *(Michael Willcocks)*

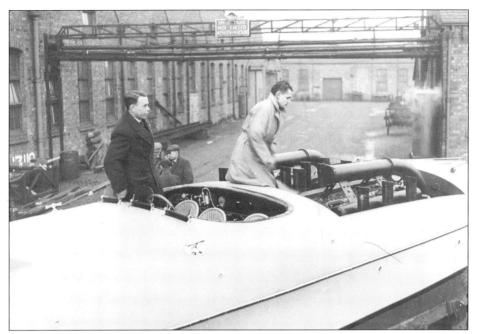

Rolls-Royce, Derby: *Miss England II* ready to run again. Willcocks in the cockpit of the boat which nearly cost him his life. The new recruit, Dick Garner, is in the engine compartment
*(Rolls-Royce Heritage Trust)*

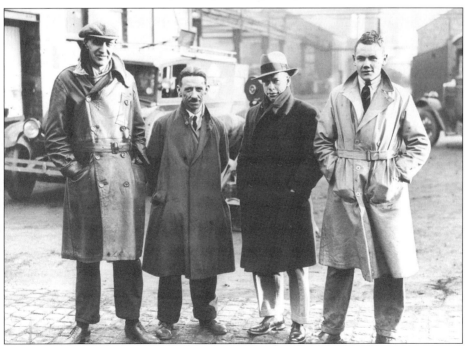

The 1931 engineering team. Second from left, Tommy Fisher, nicknamed "the midget mechanic", for his skill in scrambling inside the boat *(Rolls-Royce Heritage Trust)*

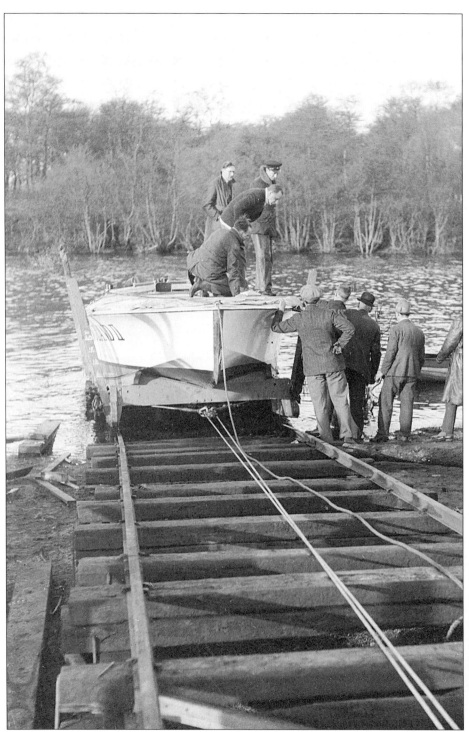
Lough Neagh, near Belfast. Kaye Don and George Eyston on the deck *(Author's collection)*

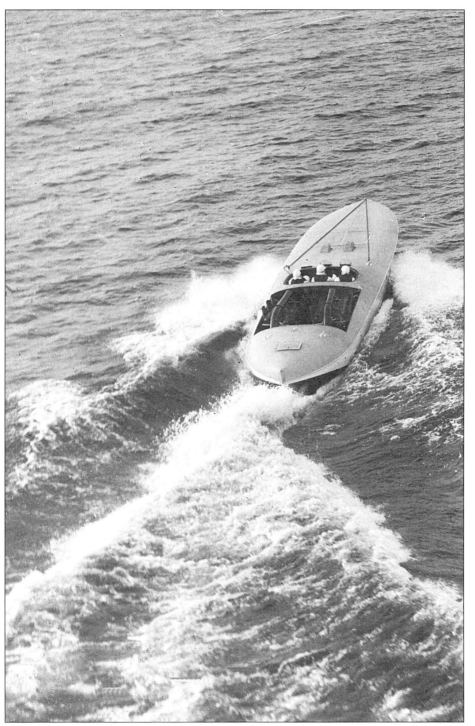

Back at speed again *(Author's collection)*

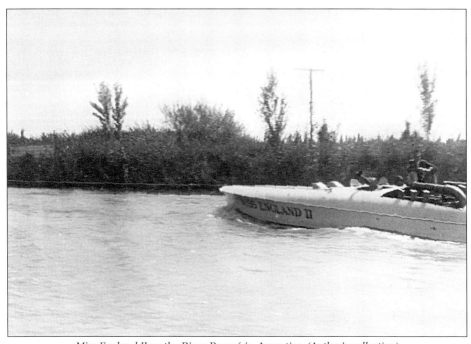

*Miss England II* on the River Paraná in Argentina *(Author's collection)*

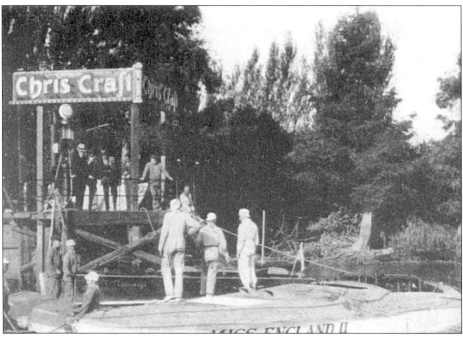

*Miss England II*'s Argentinian base was the Corporación Tiluca, local agents for Chris-Craft
*(Yacht Club Argentino)*

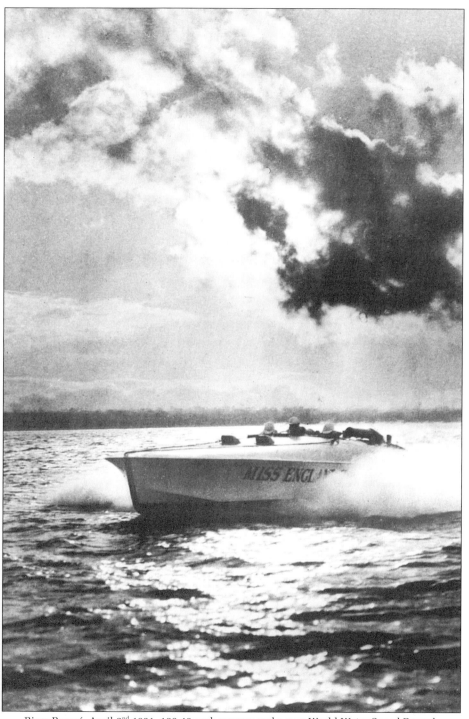

River Paraná, April 2<sup>nd</sup> 1931. 103.49 mph average and a new World Water Speed Record
*(Author's collection)*

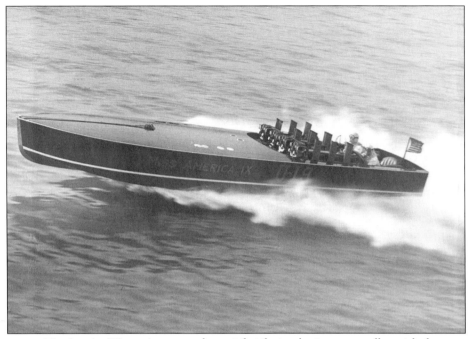

*Miss America IX's* maximum speed meant that the two boats were equally matched
*(Author's collection)*

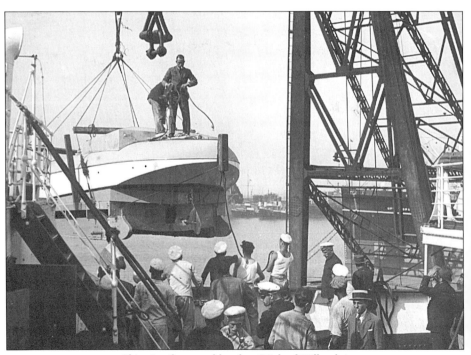

Shipping the record-breaker *(Michael Willcocks)*

*Rosario*, from which operations for clearing the river were carried out, but not with any great amount of success."

On their first four-minute trial, watched by a large crowd, Don was unable to manoeuvre the craft onto her high-speed planing trim. Worse still, weed which had escaped the drag nets blocked up the water-cooling scoop. Nine of the exhaust manifolds, situated only three inches from the fuel tanks, swiftly burned themselves out, belching clouds of smoke and starting a fire. Dick Garner promptly put this out with the onboard Kyle fire extinguisher but not before the port wooden coaming had been charred.

Willcocks described the design problems:

"Back at Cowes, when the boat was being constructed, I had asked Jimmy Ellor, the Rolls-Royce technician in charge of water-cooling: 'If the exhaust manifolds lose water, how long will it be before they get through to the petrol tank?'

"Five seconds," replied Ellor.

"Well, couldn't we have an asbestos-lined, double-surface aluminium shield right the way through?" asked Willcocks.

In the light of what happened, it was, as Willcocks noted "A good thing it had been done!"

The boat was immediately towed back to Tigre – another 'cruise' of three-and-a-half hours. The exhaust manifolds were removed and examined and it was discovered that only one of the twelve manifolds – or 'boxes' to use the slang term – was of any further use. Realising that only six spare manifolds were available from the spare 'R'-type engine, a large garage in Buenos Aires began to make up some manifolds out of sheet steel. At this stage Kaye Don, Garner and Stan Orme of Rolls-Royce unpacked the spare engine which had been stored at the Anglo Frigorifico in Buenos Aires and removed the exhaust manifolds, which Garner then took up to Tigre. As the manifolds being made up by the Buenos Aires garage would not be strong enough, the Anglo Frigorifico went all out to help the team and did a more efficient job of making up the necessary parts. According to a report written by Rolls-Royce technician Stan Orme, "These boxes were heavy, weighing twelve pounds each and were also a rough job, but more serviceable and stronger than the first firm's effort."

Back again at Tigre, repairs and preparation work went on

through the Monday night and well into Tuesday. A careful examination was made of each of the bores for scoring marks or any pieces of broken exhaust manifold. Mercifully, all the cylinders were clear and OK, except for a slight rust on the liners. The complete water system to the exhaust manifolds was next dismantled and all pipes examined for any foreign matter liable to cause a stoppage. All the system was cleared including the scoops.

A further firm asked the *Miss England II* team if they could weld up the broken boxes, claiming that they had the finest equipment and used the latest German methods of aluminium welding. The British team decided to allow them to do what they could, but only as a very last resort did they expect to have to use the boxes that had been so meticulously repaired.

Fred Cooper had the boat up on the slipway of the Tigre Yacht Club and examined her sensitive hull bottom, passing it OK. Work continued fitting up the spare aluminium manifolds. The removal and fitting of these manifolds was not an easy task, the petrol tanks having to be disconnected and moved up forward to allow the manifolds to be drawn off the studs. Having now got a complete set of manifolds, an effort was made to have the boat ready for the morning of Friday 27th March. This involved 'burning the midnight oil'.

Willcocks recalled, "Fred Cooper said to Garner and myself, 'As you've got to ride in the boat, you'd better get some sleep.' So we went to bed during the morning. I must have gone to sleep because someone came in and called me."

Everything was ready by Friday midday. After five days' delay, *Miss England II* was taken upstream for her second trial. Willcocks had asked for and obtained the participation of two speedboats to run ahead of and either side of their acceleration path which would create a wash and enable Don to get *Miss England II* up onto her planing trim. This did not work, even when the two riding mechanics ran along the foredeck in an unsuccessful attempt to use their combined weight to bring the bows down. After twelve embarrassing minutes of low-speed running, the remaining aluminium exhaust boxes burnt out.

According to the report by Rolls-Royce engineer, Stan Orme:

"The boat was immediately towed back to Tigre. It was now obvious that something drastic would have to be done. The possibilities of towing *Miss England II* at fairly high speeds was suggested for a check test on the cooling system, but Mr Cooper would not allow this to be done. Mr Cooper agreed that it was essential to fit a separate scoop to the exhaust system to overcome the climatical conditions on the Parana – tropically hot summer weather and the river water 35 degrees warmer than anything experienced on either Windermere or Lough Neagh.

"On all the trials, the discharge from the exhaust cooling was always observed to be steaming *before* the boat rose up onto her planing trim.

"A small scoop was obtained from the Chris-Craft depot, which Mr Cooper tested with a three-foot length of pipe. This scoop would deliver water over a three-foot head at approximately 12mph, the area of the scoop being slightly larger than that of the original one. This scoop was fitted on the starboard side of the boat in a similar position to that of the original on the port side. Whilst the new scoop was connected directly to the exhaust system, the old connection from the oil cooler feed was blanked off."

Saturday came and the team again cleaned the rust from the cylinders, using mineral oil. On Sunday, Fred Cooper decided to have the number 2 propeller fitted to assist Kaye Don in 'getting up on the step quicker'. When Don had asked Willcocks about the technique necessary, his riding mechanic could only reply, "No-one can tell you how to get her to plane. It's a question of touch. Try to drive as though climbing a slippery slope."

The first propeller was in a very bad condition, also through rusting, the metal being very badly eaten, giving the appearance of an acid effect on the steel. Several enquiries were made about the river water, which was a dirty brown colour, and the general opinion was that the polluted River Parana contained a certain amount of ammonia.

On Monday 30th, *Miss England II* was taken back to the Chris-Craft depot where work continued through Tuesday and Wednesday, fitting the new manifolds as they arrived. Willcocks noted that, "The new manifolds were reasonably good. But the clearances were so small for getting the nuts on because each engine was very near the hull. So we spent many hours chipping and filing and getting clearance on those nuts, fiddling and dropping several of them in the bottom of the boat. We worked day and night on this.

"During the night, we had a floodlight. Every tropical insect in the whole of Buenos Aires and the delta district came to see us. They just dropped in thousands onto the boat, attracted by the light. There were praying mantises, vast great moths and thousands of smaller insects."

In the early morning of Thursday 2$^{nd}$ April, the usual squad of newspaper reporters invaded Don's hotel room. "What are you going to show us today, Mr Don?"

"I hope to show you how records are broken, and then return to England by liner, tonight. The boat is in fine condition. So am I. Everything seems favourable this time."

The sluggish tow up to the Measured Mile at Parana began at 2 o'clock in the starlit Thursday morning so that *Miss England II* would be ready to run at sun-up. During the voyage, Garner was on board the hydroplane checking all the fastenings and the lubrication. Another Argentinean gunboat, the *Parana*, had been placed approximately five miles away, both gunboats acting as sighting points. Two Argentine Naval aircraft, the R.50 and R.60 flew directly over the course, keeping a close vigil for anything in the nature of loose driftwood that might accidentally find its way past the nets that were again stretched across the river and its many tributaries. The timing apparatus had been tested and found OK. After the usual delay and muddle for nearly an hour, Kaye Don with Willcocks and Garner set off on a third attempt.

Willcocks remembered that, "We weren't exactly without butterflies when we started to belt down the Parana. Even though they had cleared the spectator craft off the course, the danger of hitting a lump of floating driftwood at 100mph was as ever present as icebergs. We were wearing our reinforced lifejackets, but had we capsized, one or two would have been drowned. Back in England a well known racing driver called 'Sammy' Davis had advised me to cut the peak off my crash helmet, warning that if I were to hit the water, the peak would act as a fulcrum and break my neck."

With their characteristic puff of smoke and volley of flame, the 'R'-type engines started up immediately and after a short time *Miss England II* was up on the step. Don cruised around for a period and then, at 10.55am, accelerated down the course. A comparison of the six chronometers gave the average time for the two runs of 1860 yards as 42.8 seconds – 96.5mph. This was not fast enough to beat Commodore Gar Wood's record. Garner and Willcocks had great difficulty in recording any figures as they were being continually bounced out of their seats. Willcocks had blown up his air cushion too hard: "You were like a pea on a drum. You hit it and you'd bounce up and at one stage my feet were off the floorboards."

*Miss England II* was again moored alongside the Argentinean gunboat and a rapid inspection was carried out. Everything appeared OK. Garner reported that the outlet water pipe from the exhaust system kept quite cool. Kaye Don reported that he had his foot 'hard down'. So, very much doubting this, the throttle positions were checked with Don depressing the pedal. The so-called 'hard down' position was 25 degrees from full throttle. To enable the full throttle position to be obtained 'with ease', three return springs were removed, leaving only one spring on the pedal.

Whilst they were putting in a fresh supply of fuel, Kaye Don and Willcocks were taken off in a fast motor-launch to the nearby island of Cruz Colorado for lunch. "I'll never forget that lunch. It was a restaurant on stilts where they sold chickens which just about tasted like a clove of garlic. We tried to eat a bit to keep us alive, but everybody felt very sick, then I heaved my heart out from the smell of it. I thus returned to *Miss England II* with an empty stomach!"

According to a report published in 'The Herald' newspaper, "For the first time since his arrival in the country, Mr Don was not altogether imperturbable during the meal. He was obviously keyed up to a high pitch, and was frequently observed to make slight gestures of impatience, as though eager to return to *Miss England II* and get the job over. Nevertheless, he declined to permit his impatience to get the better of him, and insisted on remaining on the island until five minutes before the hour arranged for the official trials. Once aboard the motor launch on which he went back to the gunboat *Rosario*, Mr Don became his smiling easy self again ... '

Everything was now ready for a further attempt. *Miss*

*England II* began her first run at 2.55pm. A slight breeze was blowing across the course from the north, making the water choppy. During the run, the speedboat snaked rather badly but managed a time of 39.4 seconds. With a return run against the Parana's swiftly moving current timed at 40.7 seconds, the average time for the two runs of 1860 yards each was 40.05 seconds – 103.5mph. This was sufficient to snatch the World Water Speed Record from Gar Wood's grasp by a marginal 1.25mph.

After the run it was found that the cock in the gearbox had come out, accounting for much less oil in the ENV gearbox. In addition, the boat had also shipped between 60 and 80 gallons of river water in her forward section. But, mission accomplished, *Miss England II* was immediately towed back to Tigre. On landing Don was taken, shoulder high, back to the local hotel by the excited Argentineans. Those that did not carry him, cheered and clapped enthusiastically. As one Englishman observed, "These Argentineans seem to have the idea that *they* are the record-breakers."

After dinner at the Tigre Hotel and official receptions at both the Plaza Hotel and the Yacht Club Argentino, Don and Cooper hurried to the Buenos Aires dockside to catch the Blue Star liner *Avelona Star*, departure 11pm, destination England. Even here they were further cheered and enthusiastically hustled as they climbed up the gangway.

Among the minor sidelights were the measures taken by foreign press correspondents to get back to town first with the news. They had learned from experience that there were no telephones. One local representative of important British and American newspaper interests, who carried a basket of carrier pigeons out with him to the island, released them in pairs, destination Buenos Aires, with the same message in duplicate, as developments arose. The opposition had a speedboat that carried the news from Cruz Colorado to Tigre in less than half-an-hour.

Following a de-rusting of the cylinder liners, a further supply of mineral oil was placed in all cylinders for despatch purposes. Petrol and oil tanks were drained and *Miss England II* generally prepared to go on show at the British Empire Trade Exhibition. During this preparation, a sodden photograph of

Segrave was found wedged inside the bow of the boat. Someone had obviously felt that Sir Henry – or his photo – should be the first to 'cross the line'.

During the fortnight that followed, the 'victorious' *Miss England II* was on display at the British Empire Trade Exhibition. Willcocks noted that, "There were already two Scottish pipers in residence in Buenos Aires, then more were sent out there and they put on quite a good show. The English-speaking Club overlooked the Exhibition arena where they did the sword-dancing. When the pipers played 'Will ye no' come back again', there were lots of expatriate people present with tears in their eyes."

At 7.15 am on April 16th Gar Wood's mechanics lowered *Miss America IX* into the Indian River, Florida – some 5,000 miles north-west of Buenos Aires. A wind of from 6 to 8mph was blowing from the west and the runs were all made in northerly and southerly directions. After nine attempts, Gar was only able to clock 103.249mph – 0.3mph less than *Miss England II*'s new record. One week later Don arrived at London's Paddington Station. A large crowd had gathered inside and outside the station and cheers were raised when the World Water Speed Record holder stepped from the train to be received by an admiring Lord Wakefield.

Wood remained determined. On 27th April, *Miss America IX* was again lowered into the water and her twin Packard aero-engines went booming up and down the Indian River. Speeds were registered at 102.281mph, 101.657mph, 101.256mph, 100.31mph and 100.034mph. To achieve an increase of anything more than 4mph seemed to be beyond the American's reach – for the time being. Leaving his mechanics to give the boat a thorough overhaul, the Commodore went off in his motor cruiser for a week's fishing.

# 11

# The Poet

Early in May, *Miss England II* was again a tarpaulined deck-cargo on the return transatlantic journey. According to Willcocks, "We travelled back on a crowded ship called the *Conte Verde*. *Miss England II* was on the aft deck. Up for'ard there were an awful lot of people who were being returned to Italy, repatriated because of the poor conditions in South America. The ship's crew had rigged up screens to take the air right down into the hold and there was a railed-off section to let these little tiny kids get fresh air. Their arms and legs were just like broomsticks. They were starving.

"In fact the officers of the ship told me that when these people came aboard and were given ordinary ship's food, they became ill because they were not used to eating so much. To get to *Miss England II*, we had to go through the steerage quarters. These poor folk were just side by side, about three deep, like a lot of coffins. I was not happy. I didn't like that ship.

"I was glad to disembark at Genoa. I don't like a crowd. There had only been two people on the ship that could speak English and one of those died when we got to Villefranche Bay. Well, his widow was frightfully upset about this. We had had tea and meals with them during the voyage, so I offered to accompany her down, whilst they were unloading his coffin into the ferry."

*Miss England II* had arrived in Fascist Italy and, in particular, the northern lake district, to compete in a motorboat regatta organised on the 32-mile-long mountain-flanked Lago di Garda. By lifting his record by a few miles an hour, Don hoped to win the Cup presented by Commandante d'Annunzio in memory of his immortal hero – Sir Henry Segrave.

The short, bald-headed, 68-year-old Gabriele d'Annunzio, alias Prince of Nevoso, alias Gaetano Rapagnetta, alias Benito

Mussolini's arch political rival, was without doubt the most poetically colourful character to grace the shores of Italy's largest lake. During the Great War, as an aviator, he was awarded no less than two gold, three silver and one bronze medals as well as three war crosses. He had flown over Vienna dropping leaflets against the Central Powers. He flew his plane wherever danger was thickest. He was shot through the wrist and another bullet ended the sight of one eye and, for a time, blinded him completely. When the War ended, d'Annunzio was Commander of the Air Squad at Venice.

In September 1919 came the spectacular adventure at Fiume. Dalmatia, of which Fiume (present-day Rijeka) was the capital, had been taken from Austria by the Versailles Peace Treaty and made a ward of the League of Nations (the predecessor to the United Nations). Many Italians felt strongly that Fiume, on the Adriatic coast, should be – as it had once been – Italian.

D'Annunzio acted on public opinion. With 12,000 'Arditi' (shock assualt troops), a battle cruiser called the *Puglia* and two motorboat destroyers, he defied Austria single-handedly and, making what he called a 'holy entrance' into the city, occupied it. As a symbol, they took a spare anchor from the battle cruiser and set it up on a monument in the middle of the town to illustrate the permanent anchorage of Fiume to Italy. Whilst the League of Nations continued to fume, d'Annunzio ruled as an absolute dictator until the beginning of 1921. He defied the Rapallo Treaty of 1921, which gave Dalmatia its independence, and at the end of the year actually declared war on Italy! When he finally surrendered and marched out, he was received as a conqueror, not a rebel.

Soon after this, d'Annunzio took refuge in the modest hillside villa of 'Cargnacco' in a beautiful park on the Garda Riviera, with a panoramic view of one of the loveliest lakes in the world. He then proceeded to have it converted not only into his stately home but also into a national monument to be called 'Il Vittoriale degli Italiani', donating it to the nation.

During the next seventeen years, d'Annunzio, with architect Gian Carlo Maroni and a selection of fine Italian artists, sculptors and decorators would create perhaps the most extraordinary poet's 'Folly' in Europe. During this period the poet was writing 'cento e cento e cento pagine del libro segreto' ('hundreds and hundreds and hundreds of pages of the secret book').

Around a series of piazzas (squares), rose up an array of some fifteen stone buildings composed of sweeping stairways, of archways and of columns. In one hall, he had his wartime biplane suspended from the domed roof. D'Annunzio's own living quarters, which he named 'The Priory', are composed of a series of richly decorated and ornately furnished rooms, each one with its own fantastic name: The Mask-maker's Room, the Music Room, the World Map Room, the Blue Bathroom, the Leper's Room, the Way of the Cross Corridor, the Relics Room, the Writing Room of the Maimed, the Labyrinth Corridor and others. The Leper's Room was where the poet wished to be lain on his death. Several of these rooms were heavily perfumed. To run this symbol of Italian Art and Culture, the reclusive d'Annunzio organised it like a private police state, equipping it with an impressively well-armed and uniformed household of one hundred servants.

As both museum and memorial to the Fiume adventure, he had had the bows and midships of his battle-cruiser the *Puglia* dismantled piece by piece and transported to Gardone by train in some 20 wagons. He had then had it rebuilt, complete with masts, deckhouse and guns into slopes of his garden, orienting it so that it pointed across the lake in the direction of the Adriatic. He then had the ground around the *Puglia* re-landscaped with cypresses and rose-beds, whilst keeping its guns well-serviced – as if still in commission.

From as early as 1921, d'Annunzio encouraged motorboat racing on the Lake, presenting the silver Benaco Cup as a prize 'in memory of our great naval aviators'. On 10th June 1927, an Italian engineer called Attilio Bisio had officially driven d'Annunzio's *Spalato*, an Isotta-Fraschini-engined hydroplane across Lake Garda at 127kph (78.91mph). 'Il Commandante' had innocently claimed it as a new world speed record for motorboats, although by this time the record was over the 80mph mark.

In 1929, Cavaliere Edmondo Turci, a keen outboard motor-boat racing enthusiast who had competed in Paris, London, Bayonne and Venice, founded the Garda Motorboat Club with d'Annunzio as patron. Its President was Count Theo Rossi de Montelera, and among its first members was the Italian Head of State, Benito Mussolini. To encourage 'la motonautica', d'Annunzio presented a Cup 'for pure speed'. Then in 1931, poetically inspired by the heroic achievements of Sir Henry Segrave and shocked by his death, the Italian re-dedicated the cup, among the rules for which the minimum speed must be 65 knots – or 75mph.

According to Willcocks, "Getting *Miss England II* from Genoa to Garda was another thing. I knew that Italy was a very poor country, but I'd never seen such a ramshackle trailer as had been brought for us. It was more like a farm wagon. And they had thought they could use it to take a speedboat which weighed four and a half tons up over the mountains to Lake Garda.

"Eventually they put her on a train. We went at the State's expense and travelled Third Class. We arrived at the railway siding alongside Lake Garda to find that the crane would not drop *Miss England II* clear of the quayside. So we got the tugboat to put a line onto the hook of the crane and take the risk of going gently astern as the engine crane lowered out a bit. So she came down and fell in the water. I didn't like that at all but it was the only way.

"My first job was to go and inspect the slipway they had built. But it was so steep that we would never have got the boat out of the water. So I rang Fred Cooper, who advised us to find a boathouse.

"The one offered by Commodore Breda, was at Fasano; it was built on the site of an old smuggler's cave. Its only land entrance was through a dark narrow tunnel. Secrecy for the engines was still necessary. The boatwell was equipped with four pulley blocks to facilitate lifting out the hydroplane. It was also protected against gales of wind by a steel door, hinged at the bottom and pulled up by winches.

"After Buenos Aires, Garda was like Paradise. The water could be rough there, of course, but it could also be smooth. At that time of the year the water was ice-cool – and much freer of debris. In fact Tommy Fisher, of Rolls-Royce, and I used to swim there every day and go miles out."

Don declared the course ideal and publicly announced that

he hoped to raise the record to 110mph on it. Among those who made Don welcome was the British Pro-Consul in Milan, a certain Mr F.C. England!

\* \* \* \* \*

On May 13th, Don made four trial runs on the lake. Each failed, although *Miss England II* reached 100mph; the prop-shaft over-heated and had to be changed. Watching the trials, d'Annunzio remarked poetically to his secretary, "Lo spirito di Segrave e sull'aqua" – "The spirit of Segrave is on the lake." He proceeded to his 'Tower of Inspiration' and – in letters half-an-inch long – penned this remarkable document for Kaye Don:

> "Amico dal grande cuore (accettate la mia predilizione per questo epiteto inusitato, composto con uno spirito omerico, che è mediterraneo), io vivo vicino a voi ogni giorno. Invisibile, io vedo chiaramente. Silenzioso, i ascolto intensamente. Ieri il mio orrechio esperto ha indovinato il ritmo trionfante del vostro corridore. E tutta la potenza della mia anima si elevo, cantando questo canto: Sorgete, sorgete! Su, corridore! Labbra alla coppa, labbra dalla coppa: bevetela, o scagliatela giu, o scagliatela fuori bordo. Non spegnitore; e via lontano. Non salvagente et via. Un silenziatore? Via!
> Oh cuore! Oh sangue che arde! Ritorni dell'Eroe! Segrave e vicino. Altera volonta è qui. Inghilterra, rallegrati ...
> Non ricordo piu il resto.
> Vi offro la mia audace e perseverante Aquila di guerra, o Vittorioso.
> Vittoriale, 14-V-1931.
>
> Gabriele d'Annunzio.

In translation much is lost, but:

> "Great hearted friend! Suffer my predilections for this unusual epithet (voiced with Homeric spirit, which is Mediterranean), I live near to you every day. Invisible, I see clearly . Silent, I listen intensely. To-day my expert ear divined the triumphant rhythm of your racer. And all the power of my soul rose singing this song:
> Rise up, rise up! Up, runners!
> Lips to the cup, lips from the cup
> Drink or throw it down or throw it overboard
> No extinguisher and away
> No life-saver, and away

A silencer? Away!
Oh heart! Oh blood that burns!
Heroes return, Segrave is near
His proud will is here
England's good cheer ...
I forget the rest. I offer to you my audacious and persevering
eagle of war, Oh Victorious one!

Gabriele d'Annunzio'

\* \* \* \* \*

At 5.15pm, d'Annunzio, wearing the uniform of a lieuten-ant-general in the Italian Air Force, with six rows of ribbons on his tunic and brightly polished field boots, drove down to the lakeside, preceded by troops, police and boy scouts. He boarded his private Maserati-engined gunboat, carrying two torpedo tubes, two depth charges and four Hotchkiss machine guns and dashed up the lake to *Miss England II*'s boathouse. He gave three cheers to Kaye Don and told him, through an inter-preter –

"I have given your wheel my mystic touch, O Victor! If you do not break the record tomorrow, I shall die."

Not only did the poet ask innumerable questions about the speedboat, he even climbed down into its cockpit for a closer inspection. D'Annunzio then left the boatshed. Annoyed at being greeted by an applauding crowd, he picked up a stone and having thrown it at a cameraman, boarded his gunboat, with its seven-man crew. He grasped the firing handle of one of the Hotchkiss guns. A brisk broadside was fired, whistles were blown, bells clanged and bugles brayed. Gathering speed, the gunboat swept back down the lake. The poet waved his arms and cried. 'Huzza! Huzza! Huzza! O Victor, Huzza England! Huzza Don! Bravo Don!'

Don waved farewell, his right-hand grasping a magnificent silver cigarette case, ornamented with the poet's crest – an eagle – and the strange poem.

The following day, the contest was held for the Garda Shield. There were three competitors. The 4000hp *Miss England II*, the 1000hp Fiat-engined *Torino* piloted by Count Theo Rossi di Montelera, and *LIA III*, an Isotta-Fraschini-engined Baglietto hydroplane driven by Signor Antonio Becchi. *LIA III* hit a cross wave and overturned – fortunately without injury to her pilot. When *Miss England II* went round the tight course, the water was rough following a sudden thunderstorm. She was unable to match the speed set up by Count Rossi's *Torino*, whose forward rudder gave her a much better cornering. Thus, Rossi won the Garda Shield.

The other part of the Garda regatta was a series of races for smaller outboard-engined hydroplanes. The star of this show was a seventeen-year-old American driver called Miss Loretta Turnbull. Chaperoned by her parents, this white-overalled teenager arrived at Gardone with two Johnson-engined hydros. They were both called *Sunkist Kid*, because Loretta's father, Judge Turnbull was owner of the 'Sunkist' orange plantation in California.

During the Italian regatta, this charming girl took on some eighteen male pilots, fifteen of them from Italy, two from Spain and one from England. During the heats for the National Fascist Party Cup, the formidable 'home' fleet, mostly powered by the Italian Laros outboard engine, were roundly beaten by this young 'Amazon', who also set up a new 24 km record for Class C outboard hydroplanes with a speed of 65.5 km/h (40.9mph). During the regatta, d'Annunzio was cruising around in his gunboat, dancing up and down. At the finish of each race, he fired salute after salute. It was with the greatest difficulty that he was refused the request of piloting or being second engineer in *Miss England II*.

The following day, Don took *Miss England II* out again to put up his speed, but at 110mph, only 50 yards from the finishing line, the engine slowed and flames shot into the air. The supercharger had cracked, reducing *Miss England II*'s horsepower from 4,000 to only 400. As the engine was on the Secrets List, it had to be sent back to England to be repaired.

Don returned to London on May 21st. Willcocks went back to Clevedon for two weeks and married his fiancée, Helen Dunnett. Helen had recently come into an inheritance, including a motor car. She sold this so that she could accompany 'Wilkie' back to Italy – a sort of honeymoon.

With the anniversary of Segrave's death, 13th June 1931, *Miss England II* was silent in her boathouse at Fassano. She was spotlessly clean and gleaming, one garland of laurels on her proud prow, another around her steering wheel, and two vases of flowers on her for'ard deck.

Recalling this, Willcocks said: "We only had one halyard on the big flagpole of the boathouse. So Commodore Breda hoisted the Italian flag and the Union Jack together – at half mast. We took it in turns to salute."

Out on the lake, d'Annunzio paid tribute to Segrave's memory by approaching in his gunboat and dropping branches of wild olives near the boathouse. Willcocks presented the poet with the twisted steering wheel Segrave had been wrestling with at the time of his fatal accident on Windermere. He took this up to Vittoriale and placed it in the room containing Holy Relics and statues of Buddhas and Hindu gods and goddesses. It is there to this day.

Elsewhere, Cavaliere Turci arrived in London as an emissary for d'Annunzio, bringing with him 'La Coppa dell'Oltranza' (The Ultimate Cup). At a ceremony at the Park Lane Hotel, also on the 13th June, Fred May and Arthur Bray accepted this cup on behalf of the Marine Motoring Association, the governing body for motorboat racing in Great Britain. D'Annunzio's dedication read:

> I dedicate this winged Cup beyond the shocks of Chance to the severe glory and immortal example of Henry Segrave, Englishman with heart, head and hand.
>
> A bold thought stuck me during the storm when I saw the flames of the fastest vessel which has ever been admired on the Virgilian waters of Garda, as beautiful as Windermere, in the full harmony of the wave and of the heights of the elements against which Segrave fought for so long triumphantly.
>
> After Victory was held up by a sinister light from above I said: God is for Don. The depth claimed the sign. I will throw this desperate Cup to the sea. It is not a useless offering, but a grave pledge to explore the unknown, to accomplish the impossible, to demonstrate that only one thing is unlimited in the whole world: the courage of man.
>
> Since I desire to avoid the profound temptation I send the Cup to the powerful Marine Motoring Association on the eve of such a great day: of the first anniversary 13 June 1930 – 13 June 1931.
>
> A faithful and zealous presenter is Lieutenant Edmondo Turci, the

valiant driver of my Buccari motorboat ('MAS 96' – 'Memento Audere Sempre' – 'Remember Always to Dare' – 11ᵗʰ February 1918, Cross of War).

A same flame blazes from the heart of the Hero and of the Poet.

Heroism and Poetry are both resurrection.

Throw overboard, comrades, the desperate Cup of Windermere: it will sound out the depth of life and of sacrifice, of death and of immortality.

Eternal love for this name: Henry O'Neil de Hane Segrave.

Comrades, Farewell!

Vittoriale 11ᵗʰ June 1931.

Gabriele d'Annunzio de Montenevoso.

The inscription on the trophy, engraved by its creator, goldsmith Renato Brozzi, reads.

HENRY SEGRAVE
WINDERMERE THE XIII
OF JUNE MCMXXX
"How are the lads?"

Michael Willcocks had communicated the last phrase to the Italians as Segrave's first words when he had regained consciousness. Elsewhere again, members of the Windermere Motor Boat Racing Club drank a bottle of wine sent to them by d'Annunzio, whose message was that the wine "should be drunk to the immortal and glorious memory of Sir Henry Segrave and his men."

By the beginning of July, Kaye Don was back at Garda for a new trial. On July 2ⁿᵈ, just before darkness – darkness comes suddenly in a mountain-flanked lake district – a ball of flame was shooting across the lake. During this third run, Don had suddenly seen a dark object bobbing in the water ahead. He twisted the boat off its course, risking overturning, and only avoided the object by a few feet. It was a pine tree, swept down the mountainside by the snow-fed waters. Two enormous logs, weighing about a quarter of a ton each, were also found floating on the course.

On July 3ʳᵈ 1931, Don clocked a new World Water Speed

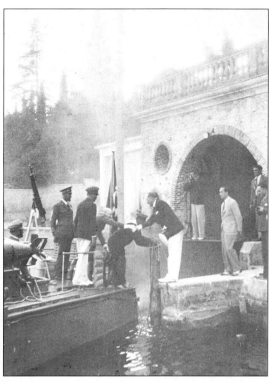

Gabriele d'Annunzio arrives in his Maserati-engined armed gunboat to inspect the legendary *Miss England II*. He is greeted by Kaye Don *(Michael Willcocks)*

Below: commemoration – June 13th 1931, one year later *(Michael Willcocks)*

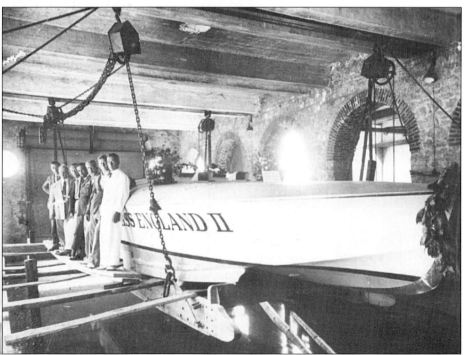

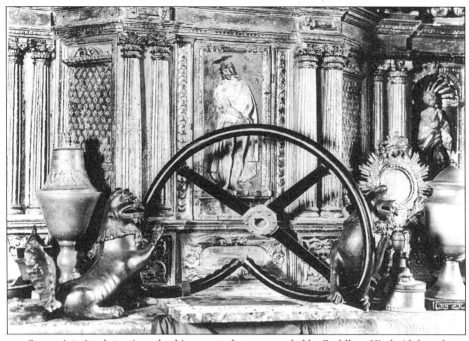

Segrave's twisted steering wheel is, even today, surrounded by Buddhas, Hindu idols and Christian icons at d'Annunzio's villa, "Vittoriale" *(Vittoriale)*

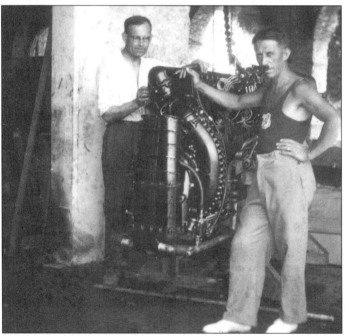

Tommy Fisher and the R-type. A cracked supercharger, then a cracked cylinder block delayed the Italian-based record attempt *(Roy Fisher)*

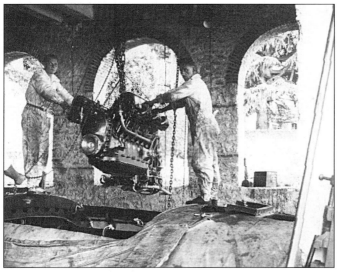

Working on the 'R'-type
*(Michael Willcocks)*

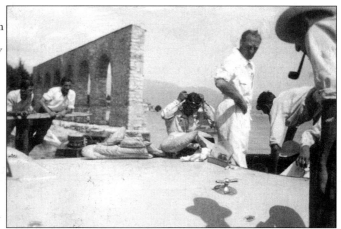

Readying for a run down Lake Garda: Kaye Don with hand in pocket, Willcocks putting on his goggles *(Roy Fisher)*

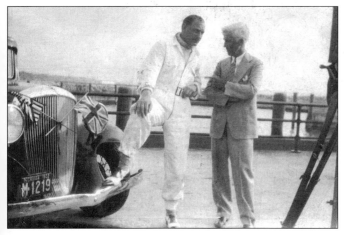

Bumper to bumper: Kaye Don and Gar Wood *(Roy Fisher)*

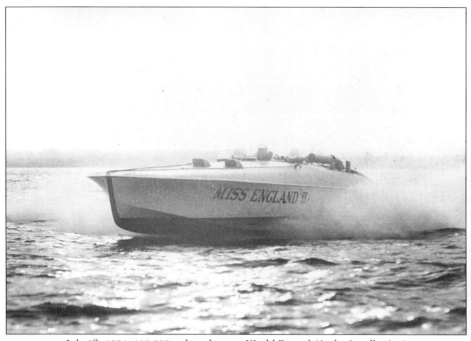

July 9th, 1931: 110.223mph and a new World Record *(Author's collection)*

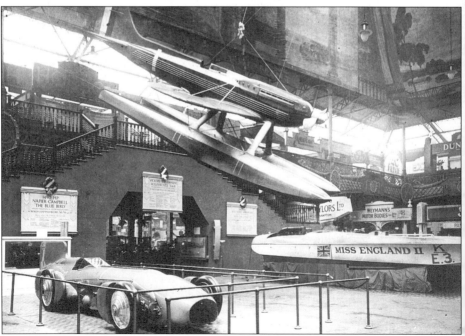

The 1931 Record Breakers: the 110mph Miss England II on show with the 245mph
Napier-Campbell car and the 328mph Supermarine S6B seaplane at the Motor Show
*(Quadrant Picture Library)*

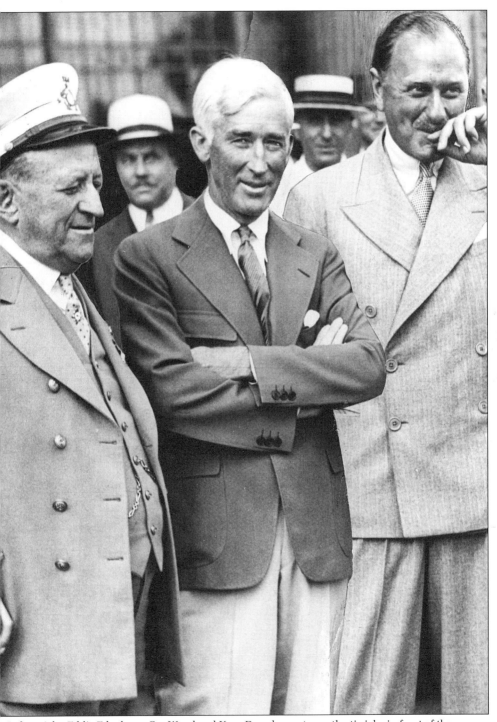

Left to right: Eddie Edenburn, Gar Wood and Kaye Don share a transatlantic joke in front of the
Press in the city of Detroit *(Richard Garner)*

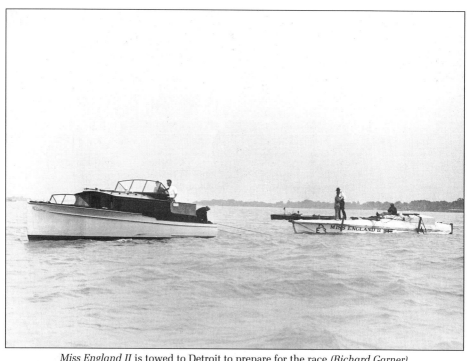

*Miss England II* is towed to Detroit to prepare for the race *(Richard Garner)*

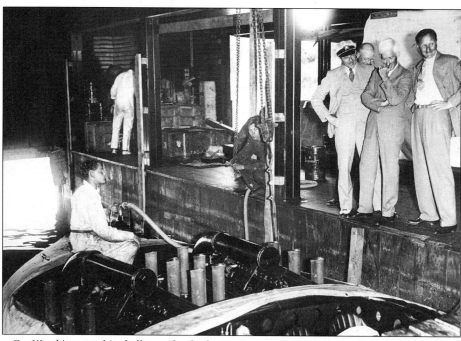

Gar Wood inspects his challenger for the first time. Dick Garner is in the engine compartment
*(Richard Garner)*

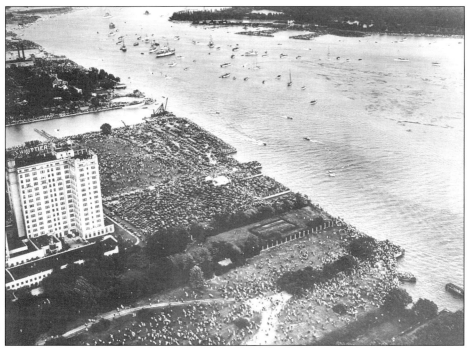

500,000 spectators gathered to watch the Harmsworth Trophy races *(Author's collection)*

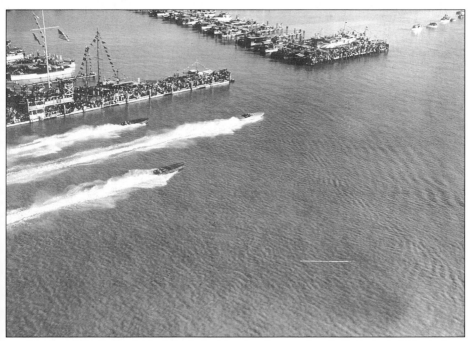

Heat One: *Miss England II* leads both the *Miss Americas* – unheard of! *(Author's Collection)*

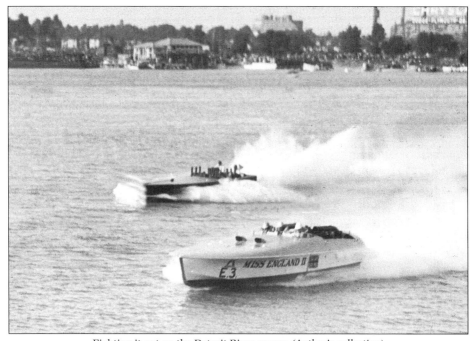

Fighting it out on the Detroit River course *(Author's collection)*

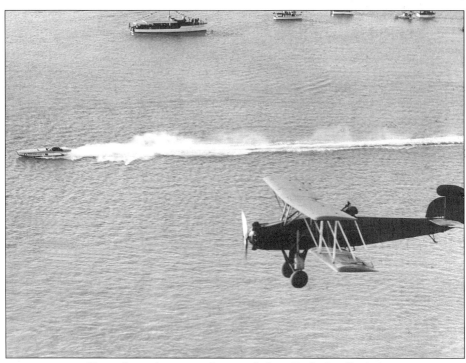

The perfect wake, as seen from an airplane *(Author's collection)*

Record of 104.9mph, with his fastest run at 109.12mph. The following day, *Miss England II* was again seen hurtling down Lake Garda, but a thunderstorm broke, the engines overheated and the boat had to be towed back to the dock. On closer inspection it was found that the port engine needed a new cylinder block. This would have to be flown in from Rolls-Royce at Derby. The pilot of the aeroplane, Captain Bailey, flew into a terrific storm and had to land at 1000ft on the edge of a precipice in the French Alps. Before long the new cylinder block had been installed and on July 9th, a magnificent day with sunshine and white clouds, the lake crowded with spectators, Don made two spectacular runs up and down Lake Garda. The first was timed at 107.879mph. The second run, at 112.569mph, created a new World Record average of 110.223mph.

D'Annunzio sent a telegram to Lord Wakefield:

> "Kaye Don has driven your wonderful boat to victory with a courage which corresponds completely to your important faith and virile expectation Stop I write many pages on this impressive Briton Stop On this world speed boat record I dedicate to you my rapid work Stop With affection for your companions, sincerely yours.
>
> Gabriele d'Annunzio."

* * * * *

Don was invited to meet Mussolini – but not before d'Annunzio had given him a magnificent reception in the grounds of his lakeside castle. Following a torchlit tour of the grounds and the *Puglia*, there was an 18-gun salute and a display of 'home-made' fireworks. Whilst the men were presented with a crate of Haig Dimple whisky and red and blue silk handkerchiefs (d'Annunzio's colours), Mrs Cooper and Mrs Willcocks each received a roll of luxurious silk mignon dress material.

Don was welcomed in Rome by 'Il Duce' and then returned to Garda where he carried out secret preparatory trials with *Miss England II* in preparation for her shipment to Detroit to challenge Gar Wood for the Harmsworth Trophy. During these trials *Miss England II* is reported to have reached an astounding 124mph.

When it was announced that *Miss England II* was to challenge for the Harmsworth Trophy, but that Willcocks would not be one of the mechanics, many people were surprised. But, as Willcocks explained, "A day or two after the record was broken on Garda, Fred Cooper rang me up and said, 'Wilkie, I'm not coming out to Detroit.' This shook me to the core.

'Why not?' I said.

'I'm not wanted,' replied Cooper

'Well that lets me out,' I said, and added, 'I'll go and see Limb at Castrol when I get back to London and say 'How d'ye do' and that's that.' "

As *Miss England II* was being towed down Lake Garda, destination the railway station at Desenzano, realising that this was the last time he would 'voyage' in this boat, Michael Willcocks wondered whether during the rest of his life he would ever experience an adventure comparable to the last, extraordinary twenty-three months.

He recalled that "Although Segrave never raced on Lake Garda, many of the local inhabitants believe that on still, moonlit nights, he speeds across the waters of the lake. The other evening, an Englishman was standing on the shore when an extra large wave broke and a boatman startled him by saying, 'E Enrico Segrave cogli occhi azzurri che passa' – 'There goes Henry Segrave, with the blue eyes'."

# 12

# Harmsworth 1931

Of all the powerboat trophies to be contested, perhaps the Harmsworth Trophy – otherwise known as the British International Trophy – can lay claim to being the oldest. It was presented in 1902 by the newspaper baron, Sir Alfred Harmsworth (later Lord Northcliffe) to promote the then lagging sport of Unlimited Motor-Launch Racing. Year after year, the contest developed such that if you built a boat that could win the Harmsworth, you probably also had the fastest boat in the world.

In the first chapter of this book, we recounted Gar Wood's winning and defending of this coveted trophy in the early 1920s. In 1928, Betty Carstairs, a flamboyant English millionairess, challenged the record with the single Napier Lion-engined hydroplanes *Estelle I* and *II*. In the consequent race, Miss Carstairs, driving *Estelle II*, hit the swell of a speedboat, flipped into the air and capsized. Both Carstairs and her mechanic Joe Harris were taken to hospital with broken ribs.

In 1929 she challenged again with *Estelle IV*, powered by three Napier Lion engines that brought the total to 3000hp. In the race, this lightweight hydroplane, with one of her Lion engines already removed to reduce violent vibrations at speed, struck a submerged log at 70mph and had to be retired.

In 1930 a new *Estelle IV* and *Estelle V* challenged three *Miss Americas*. Had *Miss England II* not crashed on Windermere, Segrave would have taken her out to Detroit to join with Betty Carstairs in her attack. As it was *Estelle V*'s fuel tanks disintegrated, the engine caught fire and the pilot had to retire on the first heat, then the *IV* retired because of exactly the same problem in heat two.

Betty Carstairs could not make a fourth challenge in 1931. "I have tried for the Harmsworth Trophy three times without success. I cannot afford another attempt." It thus remained for Kaye Don to carry the flag.

For his defence, Wood held two *Miss Americas* on stand-by – numbers *VIII* and *IX*, to be driven by himself and his brother George. Each boat was built of mahogany, measured 28ft long and was powered by two 12-cylinder Packard engines, developing a total of 2,280hp against *Miss England II's* 3,380hp. Although *Miss America IX* had shown herself capable of a World Speed Record of 102mph at Miami, to give her the edge of speed in a race which promised to be closely fought, Wood sent her engines to the Packard Motor Car Company to have superchargers fitted that would give a maximum of 3,000hp and a potential 115mph.

He also experimented with a heavier bow rudder on the *IX* to help her round the turns but, finding that this made her uncontrollable, changed back to the smaller rudder.

On Wednesday August 12th 1931, Kaye Don left Waterloo Station, London to arrive at Southampton Docks in time for the departure of the White Star Liner, *Majestic* for America. Two days later, *Miss England II* and her mechanics left on the *Duchess of Bedford*, bound for Detroit.

'Dick' Garner, had stayed on with the boat and been joined by Roy Platford, also of Rolls-Royce. Garner recalled, "We shipped her out from Liverpool on a pretty grey and grim morning. On the Atlantic crossing there were a large number of young American and Canadian students , university types who'd been doing their Grand Tour of Europe, so we had a wonderful time.

"I can remember that the ski champion of Canada was with them, and as we went down the St Lawrence, he insisted on walking along the deck-rail at about 4 o'clock in the morning. He must have walked ten yards before we finally lost our nerve and pulled him off!

"*Miss England II* was launched and towed across to Edsell Ford's boathouse. Although it has been said that Fords were behind us because Packards were backing Gar Wood, I personally thought their hospitality was a fairly generous gesture. In fact, the original Henry Ford came round to our boathouse and it was a great honour to meet such an ordinary, keen, quiet type of American. You wouldn't have guessed he'd founded such a vast Empire.

"We had a manager over there by the name of W.D. 'Eddie' Edenburn. He was Secretary of the American Power Boat Association and Chairman of the Race Committee of the Yachtsmen's Association of America, which controlled the British International Trophy races. Eddie knew everybody in America. The Harmsworth Trophy was an enormous event at that time – so I think everybody wanted to help.

"In 1931, Detroit was quite some city. It was the days of Prohibition. We were also pestered to death every night, because there would be different women knocking every half-an-hour and it was a most unpleasant business. So I finally went and lived on a cruiser that somebody loaned us at the Detroit Yacht Club and we slept on board in preference to that hotel.

"We didn't see a gangster fight, but we saw plenty of people paralysed through hooch, the nickname for illicitly distilled alcohol. Fortunately we were with people who knew where to go to get a good drink in the Motor City. There was a place called 'The Pioneers' Club' on Jefferson where, although it took you about ten minutes to be vetted at the door, once you were in you had all the good English booze you wanted. You didn't have to risk drinking any of the bootleg hooch. However, we'd go out on the city at night and several times we went to 'The Blind Pig', which was a hooch joint, just to have a look. But compared with today, Detroit was quite a pleasant city.

"Our first job was to get *Miss England II* unplugged, cleaned and all systems tested out to make sure there was no damage. We'd run the engines in the dock. It was a well-equipped dock in a fairly well-secluded place on the Detroit River. We had a fireman and a policeman on 24-hour watch, so we were well guarded."

Before long, Kaye Don had invited Gar Wood down to the boathouse. After taking a good look at *Miss England II*'s lines, he commented, "It's a sturdy enough boat and it must be good or it couldn't have reached the speed it did in setting its record. They have strengthened up the step but to me it doesn't seem to have enough buoyancy up forward. We'll find out later just how good she is!"

Apart from their love of speed, in terms of personality and racing experience, Wood and Don were two very different types.

Gar Wood, 'The Commodore', was a wiry, white-haired 50-year-old Detroiter, whose gruff and rugged manner often betrayed the fact that he was the millionaire head of a vastly successful hydraulic hoist and boatbuilding concern. He owned 'Grayhaven', a large private mansion built of Georgian Bay granite on the banks of the St Clair River. Enter it and you might hear a music box, a synchronised organ-and-piano device, playing in the background. Its tallest pipe went from the ground floor to the attic. Revolving lights were set mysteriously behind panes of frosted glass in the ceiling, changing the colours from half darkness to purple, then to violet, then to pale rose. There was a massive indoor swimming pool and a lounge capable of seating 75.

An odd little tower jutting from Wood's winter home in Miami Beach enclosed a finely equipped observatory, including a chair with a hydraulic hoist that enabled the observer to sit comfortably at whatever angle he surveyed the heavens. He had car radios – a rare thing in the early 1930s – in each of his nine automobiles, which included custom-built Packards and Duesenbergs. He also owned a $35,000 aerial yacht. With a total of thirty years' experience in racing powerboats, Gar Wood had become a master in the art of skidding a high-speed hydroplane round the buoys. He was soon to be nicknamed 'The Grey Fox' on account of his wily racing strategies.

In contrast, Kaye Don, now 30, a company director, was always well-spoken and always immaculately dressed. His hobbies included theatre-going and golf, and he was completely free of superstition. His ten years' experience and success in racing motor-cars up to 130mph around the treacherous bankings of Brooklands track, near Weybridge, Surrey, had earned him the title of 'King of the Concrete'. His experience in racing boats was still extremely limited. Knowing every solid bump on Brooklands track was not the same as having a mariner's encyclopaedic knowledge of the ever-changing whims and currents of the Detroit River.

The supercharged Packards for *Miss America IX* had only arrived five days before the first heat and whilst Wood was

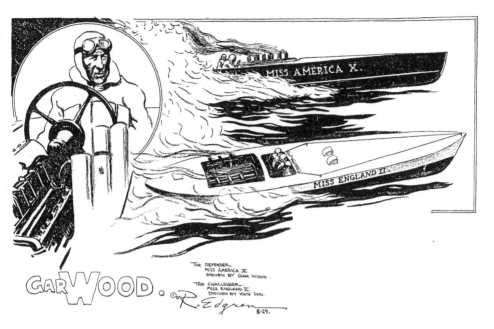

A pro-Wood contemporary cartoon

installing and testing them at Algonac, his home at the upper end of Lake St Clair, Don was putting *Miss England II* through trials over the Trophy course, proving a surprise to the increasing number of fans, who began to line the river every morning at daybreak.

According to Dick Garner, "We probably covered 100 nautical miles in practice. Our starting point, going for the Line, was directly opposite Grayhaven, where Gar Wood had his pits. From there he would be driving his *Miss Americas* out from his dock entrance at the beginning of Heat One. So we practised how long it would take us to get onto the step and hit that Line flat-out. We did this with stopwatches. I had a stopwatch and two starting watches on the deck as well. If I remember rightly, we reckoned our time was 12 seconds from Grayhaven to over the Starting Line flat out. 'Hump' speed was 50-60mph and we reached 100-110mph in six to eight seconds, which gave us the four to six remaining seconds at full throttle towards the Line. We must have practised this at least a dozen times.

"After hitting the Line, you'd got a relatively short run before you throttled back for the Belle Isle buoy, which was the sharp-

93

est bend on the course, where the river narrows just before the bridge, and where our boat became rather unstable. Coming into it fairly fast, Kaye Don got this fairly well mastered but we skated a lot and you could feel her skidding sideways. Then we had a fairly long straight run with a relatively easy left-hand bend and a fairly wide sweep past Grayhaven, out into Lake St Clair, so we could keep the boat going reasonably well, without undue side-slipping, then back down another fairly reasonable bend, just before Grayhaven and then straight for the line again. The difficult bit was going fast enough over the Line and being able to slow down enough to get round the Belle Isle corner."

On September 3rd Don decided to curtail his preliminary runs to avoid mishaps which had befallen Harmsworth Trophy challengers in previous years.

The Detroit River was swept by the edge of a storm on September 5th; the storm circled over Lake Superior and, by Saturday afternoon, the wind had hauled round into the south-west. A south-wester on the Detroit River is directly against the current and piles up short, choppy seas in which any high-speed hydroplane could only survive by a miracle. At the easterly end of the course, where the wind had a mile sweep off the Canadian shore, there were waves about 3ft long and 26-28 inches in height. although it was the first day for the scheduled races, Kaye Don asked for a postponement, which Wood readily granted.

By the evening of Sunday 6th September, the wind had hauled round to the south-east and the course, while not smooth, was not sufficiently rough to endanger both the hydroplanes. *Miss England II* was towed out to the main dock of the Detroit Yacht Club and her crew calmly waited the preparatory five-minute gun.

An estimated half to three-quarters of a million spectators had gathered to watch one of the major sporting events in the North American Calendar. Dick Garner said, "I was quite impressed by the crowds, but at the same time you were so tensed up that you really didn't notice that sort of thing. When you knew you'd got to go out across the river and be sure that everything was thoroughly warmed up, with just enough fuel in the tanks, the magnetos checked, and the time and tappet settings checked, you had little time to think about applause."

The course was 5 miles around and had to be covered six times, making a distance of 30 nautical miles. The 5-minute gun was fired at 6.25pm; *Miss England II* was towed out into the course, her engines were started and run-up procedure began. It had been the Wood plan to overtake Don at the first Belle Isle buoy, heading him off and giving *Miss England II* the wash of one of the *Miss Americas*. But in Dick Garner's words, "We made such an immaculate start, hitting the line under two seconds behind the starting signals, that we were first over by a matter of three or four lengths and we led all the way round."

Not that America did not try to overtake England. As Gar Wood later commented, "To pass him, I'd have to cross one or two hills of water in his wake. To pass him on the turns, I'd not only have to go faster than his boat, but I'd have to take his water. His boat had plenty of Vee and it threw up plenty of water. It was fine water, though, almost like steam. It didn't bother us much."

On the second lap, as the boats wheeled around the sweeping turn at the lower end of the course, Wood summoned forth all his experience and deep-rooted knowledge of the Detroit River to manoeuvre into a favourable position. As Don slowed to negotiate the bend, Wood nodded to his mechanic, Orlin Johnson, to give the *IX* the gun. With exhaust pipes belching forth fumes and smoke, she crept up on the outside, but as she swerved in near the shore, she encountered rough water and started to buck like a perverse bronco. Wood had only one recourse – to slow down before his boat pounded itself to pieces.

At the end of the third lap – distance 15 miles – *Miss England II* was nearly three-quarters of a mile ahead of the *Miss America* boats. As was generally expected, she skidded badly at the turns and lost much ground, but her superior speed on the straights made up for the leeway. At the end of the race, *Miss England II* was 42 seconds and about a mile ahead and her average speed for the course was 89.913mph, with her fastest lap at 93.017mph – while *Miss America IX*'s highest was 91mph on one lap.

The two boats came in to the wildest of cheering and after the two drivers had posed for photographers in the setting sun, Wood shook his hands in a gesture of despair and commented,

"The cup has been getting mildewed here. It's about time it went back!" Dick Garner recalled, "After winning that first heat, we were very elated, but that evening we did not go out on the town. One of us always stayed the night in the boathouse – we had a bunk down there as well. I think I may have gone to bed that night because I'd got to race the following day."

After the first heat, the Wood team discovered that *Miss America IX*'s Packard engines were a little off balance and had given her hull such a pounding that two of her side planks had split and two gasoline tanks cracked. By the following day, they were busy making repairs and re-adjustments. They'd got new planks and equipment from Algonac, were putting them in, taking out the tanks and soldering them up.

While this was going on behind the scenes, the countless spectators were being entertained by the second annual Dodge '16' 50-mile Sweepstakes race for no less than thirty-four stock boats, many of which were Dodge 14ft Vee-bottomed runabouts. Horace Dodge, millionaire head of the Dodge truck concern, offered one to Betty Carstairs, who was present as a spectator on his yacht. The 'little lady' declined to drive it and instead offered the helm to her guest Michael Willcocks. But the race was won by Frank Wigglesworth of Boston, who repeated his victory of the previous year driving *Miss Aldine* at an average speed of 32mph and winning $1,600. Willcocks finished seventh in his boat.

Meanwhile, back at the Gar Wood boatwell at Grayhaven, with one hour to go before the start of Heat Two, they were refilling the repaired petrol tanks, when they discovered that one of them still had a 6-inch crack in it. Wood is reported to have said, "We won't be able to start in time" – and telephoned the Judge's stand to ask for a postponement.

"The International Commission was called to Commodore Wood's boathouse at about 5 o'clock and advised that the Commodore desired a postponement of half an hour or 45 minutes, that repairs might be made to the fuel tank. The Commission immediately set out by boat to confer with Kaye Don." Don's reply – "No. We are all ready to go, our oil is hot, and that's that I'm afraid" – was no superficial one.

In starting *Miss England II* before a run, it was necessary to have a period of about 1 hour 15 minutes so that all the lubricant for the engines might be heated to the proper temperature, before it was placed in the powerplants. By the time the lubrication oil had been replaced, the race could not have been started before 6.15pm and, with sunset at 6.56, it was getting pretty close to dusk, which furnished' further hazards. Don also argued that the USA still had one boat left in the race – *Miss America VIII*.

Going back into Harmsworth history, Gar Wood had consented to postponements from two hours to two days for the challenging boat in the years 1921, 1922 and 1928. In the whole decade of his holding the Trophy, he had never previously asked for a postponement. According to the Associated Press, Gar Wood is quoted as expressing his annoyance at not even being allowed 15 minutes by saying, "When they told me that I could not have it, I made up my mind I would show Don a trick or two."

With only twenty minutes to go before the start, there was no time to empty the tank. They were not able to reach it with a blow-torch before the benzol fuel had begun to leak. So they decided to risk turning it over and soft-soldering it with an electric iron with the fuel still inside, taking a long chance on an explosion which could have blown the *Miss Americas* and their twenty-man team to smithereens.

One of Wood's best mechanics, John Brewer, shinned under the decks, scraped off the solder, took the hot iron and began to re-solder up the crack, while everyone stood by with bated breath. When Brewer was hauled out half-suffocated from the effect of the fumes, Orlin Johnson, Wood's ever-faithful riding mechanic, climbed in to finish off the job. It was completed, safely, just under five minutes before the start.

Meanwhile, *Miss England II* was waiting. Dick Garner recalled what happened next: "So off we went out into Lake St Clair again, ready for the start. Our starting point was where the Wood boys came out from Grayhaven, about 200 to 300 yards away. We were gently cruising around, looking at our watches, ready for our time start technique. All of a sudden, we saw Gar's boat shoot out and go for the Line. Kaye Don put his foot down and went after him without a word. I slammed him in the ribs and yelled 'No, No, No!' But I'm afraid he took no notice. You see, we were much too early, but he just literally roared after

Gar Wood and I think he was so mad at being behind that he rather missed what he was aiming at."

*Miss America IX* came down the course on the outside, veering in a bit as she neared the Line, motors throbbing and exhaust pipes belching forth smoke and flames. Nearer the shore came Don at a terrific speed. Two seconds apart, they thundered away together, Wood beating the gun by 9.56 seconds and Don by a little more than 7.26 seconds. Rules stated that if the boat crossed the Line more than five seconds ahead of the starting time, the boat was to be automatically disqualified.

On the inside, Wood began to take the turn in the fashion that years of experience had made possible. He clung to the buoys and Don swept round him, throttle almost wide open. He hit *Miss America IX*'s wash in front of the Little Boat Harbour, climbed the wave, teetered precariously for a second, then overturned, breaking *Miss England II*'s back.

Dick Garner stated, "We went into the beam of Gar's wash. If we have to be quite honest, I could see this happening so I drew my knees from under the dashboard and slammed the engine coolant controls wide open. I let go everything and waited for the crunch. I rolled myself into a ball, flew through the air quite happily. The next thing I knew, I surfaced, had a look round and saw the boat upside down."

In a contemporary interview, Don elaborated, "The boat went into a skid, which I corrected, but the next instant she went into the air, completed a turn and dived into the water. Neither of my mechanics suffered any serious injury. Dick Garner, who rode on my right, was thrown across me and clear of the boat, and Roy Platford on my left, sank with the boat. As we went down and down into the water, the first thought which flashed through my mind was whether we were inside the boat or not."

Dick Garner bruised his shoulder, Roy Platford was knocked unconscious and Kaye Don escaped with a wrenched knee.

While tenders rushed out to *Miss England II*, *Miss America IX* went on until flagged down. When *Miss America VIII* completed the first lap, Gar waved to her driver, his brother George, to continue on, only to prevent the course from becoming congested and to allow an attempt to be made to tow *Miss England II* ashore. The boat sank before aid could reach her.

The Racing Committee's ruling was: "The seventeenth running of the British International Trophy resulted in *no match*. The challenger was eliminated from the match through disqualification at the start of the race through crossing the line 7.26 seconds ahead of the start flag, ball and gun ...". In British Team Manager Eddie Edenburn's words, "It had been a pyrotechnical display of everything that a race shouldn't be."

There had even been accidents among the crowds. When more than 175 spectators on the temporary bleachers adjoining the Waterworks Park rose to their feet as the starting gun sounded for Heat Two, a sharp crack was heard and 40 feet of the dock sloped off into the water, only 5 ft deep but with a soft and treacherous mud bottom. Other spectators rushed to the aid of floundering men, women and children. The only spectator missing was a three-year-old boy called Nelson Pattison. Although police dragged the river that night, they failed to find the little boy's body.

Alongside this, five Canadians returned from the race and were rescued in Lake St Clair after their speedboat capsized. They were picked up by the yacht *Clarinda*, owned by Colonel Jesse G. Vincent, Vice-President of the Packard Motor Company.

When the British and American newspapers appeared next morning, the world read how Commodore Garfield Wood had been a 'bum sport' for totally disregarding the ethics of the game. The race race had been won by deliberately tricking Mr Kaye Don over the Line before the Starting Gun, so disqualifying them both, so that Mr George Wood might legally cruise around the course at a safe 60mph – and so that America might win the equalising heat.

# 13

## Fiasco

To this day, the controversy continues as to exactly what happened because there are so many differing and contradictory reports. To support the accusation, there is the original Associated Press report on what Gar Wood said: "When they told me I could not have it, I made up my mind I would show Don a trick or two ... I planned the start. I would be over the line first, even if I were a minute ahead of the gun and if Don wanted to follow me that was his business."

The 'Detroit Times' reported him as saying: "Sure I'm happy. I asked for a postponement of the start because ... my request was denied and it made me angry. If I could have the tank repaired in time ... I was coming down the river and make a false start purposely. When I did, Don likely would follow me ... if Don wanted to play that way with me, all right. I figured I could outsmart him and you know what happened." One report went even further: "From a source close to Wood, it was learned that the entire plot to trick Don of victory if possible, was planned in the boathouse of the *Miss America* boats an hour before the race. The informant, who demanded that his identity remain secret, said 'The race worked out just as was planned there an hour before the race.' Asked if the plot was designed after Don had denied Wood a 45-minute delay, he said 'No, it was long before that.'"

In Dick Garner's opinion: "There is no doubt whatsoever that Gar Wood deliberately came out to tempt us over the Line because George Wood didn't come out with him. George Wood went over that Line *25 seconds late*."

The Press had a field day of anti-Wood comments: "Wood is quoted as saying that he played a very scurvy trick on Kaye Don, his competitor whom he knew he could not beat." And: "If the

Briton was not considerate, that was no excuse for Wood to resort to deceit to bring about the defeat of his opponent. If these contests cannot be conducted on a plane that is a credit to the sportsmanship of both countries, they might better be abandoned. Americans generally will hope that the race committee will declare it to be 'no match'. Americans do not want trophies that are not fairly won." And: "Feeling in many motorboating circles over this matter is very bitter."

Then there were those reporters like Damon Runyon, who admitted Wood's trickery, then justified it: "This idea that seems to be generously fostered by many of our sports scribes and editorial writers, too, that Americans are invariably wrong in the matter of ethics and sportsmanship, and that foreigners are always right, gives me a severe pain in the neck. Just at present, the boys are putting the blast on our Mr Gar Wood, that speedboat shark, for luring Mr Kaye Don, of England, across the Starting Line ahead of the gun in the race for the Harmsworth Trophy. In fact, some of the lads are quite red in the face with indignation over this incident, though they may be surprised to learn that many old subscribers, after hearing Mr Wood's explanation, do not share in their feeling ... Mr Gar Wood's idea was, of course, that both his canoe and the English raft would be disqualified for copping a sneak and Brother George would dodder along and win the heat. It happened that Mr Don's boat, hastening after Mr Gar Wood, got caught in the wash of the American craft and went down to Davy Jones' locker, but that disaster wasn't included in Mr Gar Wood's plot. It just happened.

"Well, the ensuing wuff-wuff was terrific. No-one thought of suggesting that Mr Kaye Don might have pulled a boner in letting Mr Gar Wood draw him out in that fashion. After all, Mr Don must have known that it was no start until the gun popped. He could have waited for the signal, Mr Gar Wood would have been disqualified and Mr Don could then have gone on and licked Mr George Wood like breaking sticks. Mr Don is getting all the sympathy and Mr Gar Wood all the abuse, but I never heard of any condolences for a base runner who got caught napping off first by a crafty pitcher."

One commentator went 'over the top': "The pro-Britishers who are abusing Wood would very likely be the ones to find some technical error in the Battle of Bunker Hill and petition Congress to give the old USA back to the Crown."

Gar Wood himself contradicted statements that he had tricked Don: "We wanted to get over the Line first. I had ridden in Don's wash for thirty miles on Sunday afternoon and I knew what it was like. We felt that if we had got away first we'd have a chance to keep the lead." Wood wept as he discussed the statements attributed to him after the race, "I've been racing for years and we've done the best we could to carry the American flag on our boats in a sportsmanlike way. I don't know how this misunderstanding can be rectified. I've just talked with London over the telephone and they don't seem to understand at all what happened over here." Wood broke down at this stage and said he could not talk about it any more.

Then, to complete the controversy, in an interview he gave to the British newspaper 'The Daily Mirror', Wood recounted: "I was bound and determined to lead him next day – and prove that *Miss America IX* could make more than 110mph. Don wanted to arrange three lanes, one for himself, one for my brother and one for me. "We'll each have our own lanes up to the starting line and we'll not deviate from them."

"OK," I replied.

"Another thing. I'm going to hit that line at 110mph, and we ought to have everything cleared, for God help anybody that gets in my way."

"OK," I said. "I'll hit the line at top speed too. But watch the time balls to see you don't get away ahead of time."

"Don't worry," he replied, "I've been practising."

"We got into our channel with about two minutes to spare before the starting gun. 'Get ahead of him,' I instructed Johnson 'and stay ahead of him. If he's going to hit the line at 110mph, so will we.' My watch wasn't running, nor was Johnson's. The terrific pounding of the day before had affected both timepieces, but we weren't worried. We relied on Kaye Don to give us the time. There was nothing wrong with his watch. He'd been practising for two weeks to make that line on time, and if we were a second or two ahead of him, that was OK. We started when Don started. 'Keep a hundred feet ahead of him,' I said. Johnson obeyed orders. Don speeded up. We speeded up. He put on more speed. So did we. I wasn't watching the time balls. I

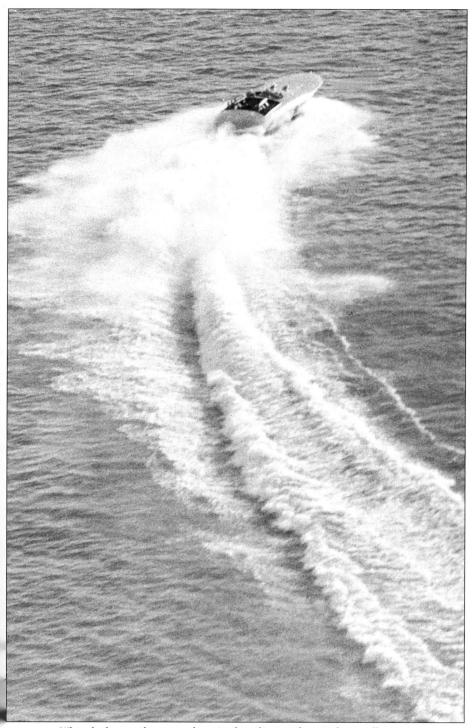

What she lost on the turns, she gained on the straights *(Author's collection)*

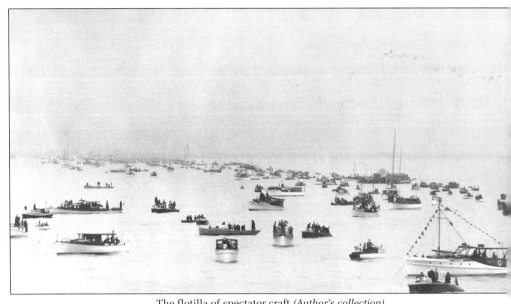

The flotilla of spectator craft *(Author's collection)*

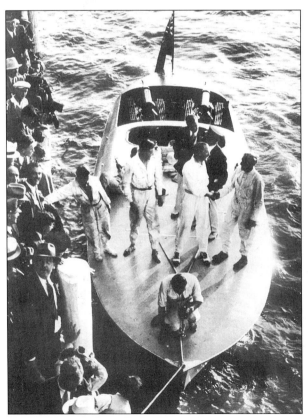

Wood congratulates Don on winning Heat One, with a heat speed record of 89.9mph *(Richard Garner)*

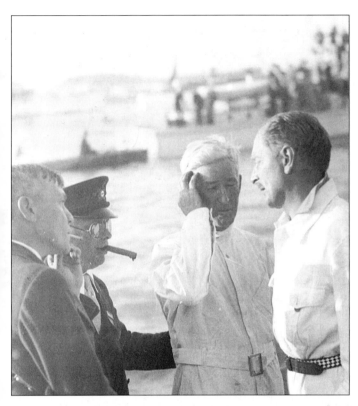

Don versus Wood ...
something's not right
(Richard Garner)

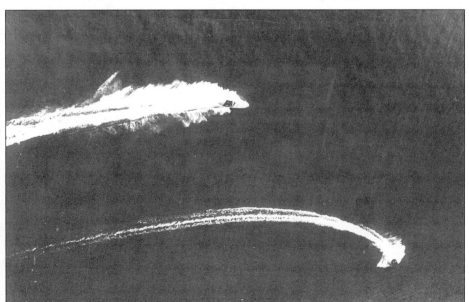

*Miss America IX* leads *Miss England II* over the line before the starting gun ... *Miss England II* just
before she capsized *(Author's collection)*

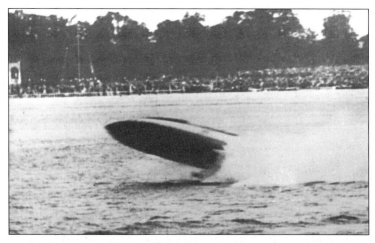

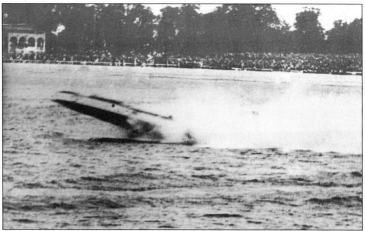

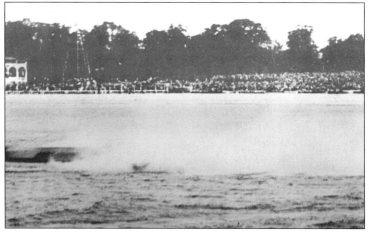

Stills from ciné film of the second flip of *Miss England II* in fifteen months
*(Author's collection)*

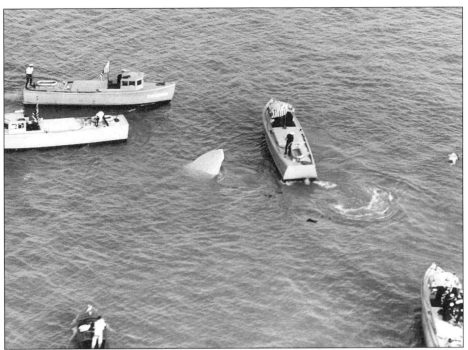

US Coastguards hurry to rescue the British crew *(Author's collection)*

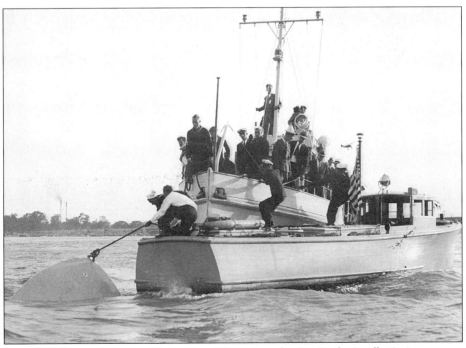

Once again in tow, this time by a US Coastguard cutter *(Author's collection)*

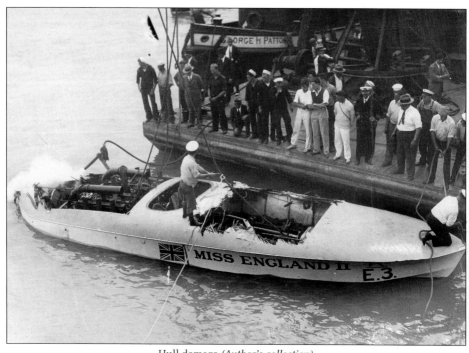

Hull damage *(Author's collection)*

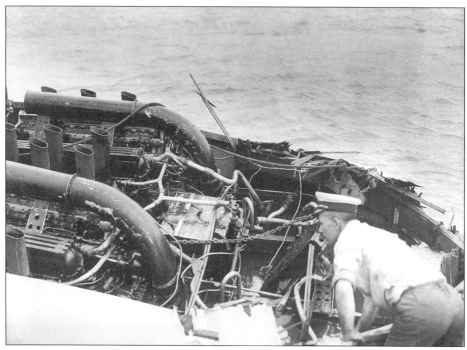

Engine damage *(Author's collection)*

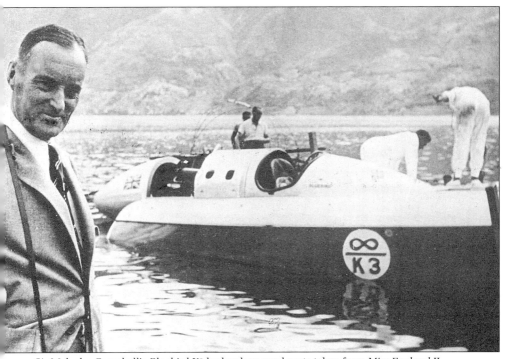

Sir Malcolm Campbell's *Bluebird K3* hydroplane used parts taken from *Miss England II*
*(Leo Villa)*

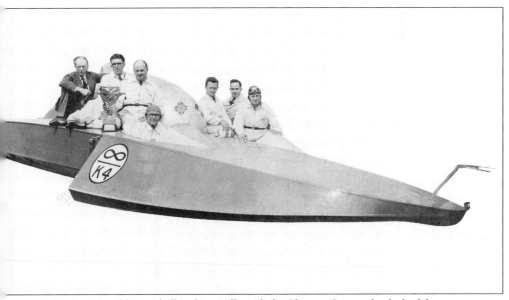

A victorious Donald Campbell and Leo Villa with the Oltranza Cup on the deck of the
*Bluebird* prop-rider *(Leo Villa)*

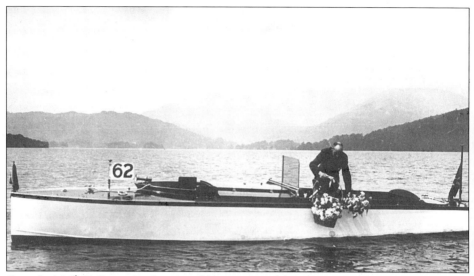

Every June 13th, T. Cooper Pattinson would motor out to White Cross Bay in his Wolseley-engined Saunders motor launch *Peggy* and lay two commemorative wreaths on the water – one for Segrave and the other for Halliwell *(T. Cooper Pattinson)*

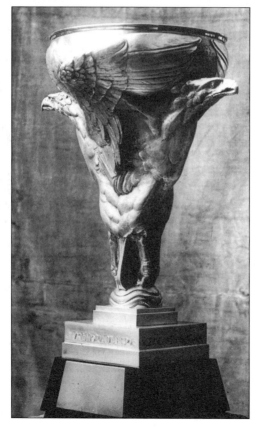

The Oltranza Cup *(Vittoriale)*

wasn't watching anything but Don. At the starting line, I was still one hundred feet ahead of him and I was going good."

Gar Wood went to great lengths to try to rebuild his image. The Duplex Oil Company of Buffalo, New York, published a small pamphlet on the contest.

Another version of the race was to appear in the biography 'Kaye Don, the Man', written by James Wentworth Day and published in London in 1934, whilst yet another version was to appear in '25 Years with the Speedboat Kings' (in reality, a biography of Gar Wood) by James Lee Barrett and published in Detroit in 1939.

But as H.G. Salsinger wrote in the 'Detroit News' – "Reams and reams will be written about the Harmsworth Trophy race of 1931. Some will be complimentary, others derogatory ... Is a motorboat race, such as the Harmsworth Trophy, a sporting event or a commercial proposition? The answer to the question will decide the issue. If it is a sporting venture then Gar Wood may be condemned; if it is a commercial proposition , then his work must be highly commended."

Shortly after dawn on September 8th, Chief Carpenter's Mate R.I. Gleason, of the US Naval Reserve gunboat, *Dubuque*, volunteered his services as diver and before long had located *Miss England II*. She was raised at 2.30 in the afternoon – for the second time in her extraordinary career. Although her deck and stern were ripped open like matchwood, it was found that the underbody of the hull was undamaged.

That same evening, George Wood drove *Miss America VIII* around the course for three laps until he was stopped and then claimed the Trophy under the rules, protesting against the first decision of the Committee which had declared it no race. Gar Wood was one of the few spectators. Dick Garner wrote: "And that unfortunately was the end of our attempt to win back the Harmsworth Trophy. We had to leave Detroit fairly soon, because we were due to show our hydroplane – now smashed up – at the Canadian National Exhibition."

Kaye Don arrived at Toronto by aeroplane from Windsor and received a tumultuous welcome. He was given a Civic welcome at the City Hall by Mayor Stewart, and afterwards entertained at luncheon by the Empire Club. Dick Garner was also there: "I did a bit of motorboating in Toronto with a large Johnson outboard on a B-Class boat. I roared around to the point where I flipped it quite happily. You see, I had decided that I had better have the distinction of flipping with two boats in one year. I succeeded."

It was then decided to build a third *Miss England*. So although, in February 1932, Gar Wood had regained the record by a margin of 1.44mph, only five months later, *Miss England III*, with Don at the wheel, answered with a new record of 119.81mph on Loch Lomond, Scotland. The Rolls-Royce engined hydroplane was then shipped out to Lake St Clair Michigan, where Don again challenged 'The Grey Fox' in his quadruple-engined 6,400hp *Miss America X* for the 1932 Harmsworth Trophy races. But *Miss England III* suffered mechanical failure in both heats – leaving Gar Wood once again unbeaten. A couple of weeks later *Miss America X* averaged a new World Water Speed Record of 124.86mph on Lake Michigan – an increase of 5.16mph.

This ought to have been the signal for Don to hit back, either using the *III* or with a new *Miss England IV*. But Lord Wakefield of Hythe decided to pull out of powerboat sponsorship 'for personal reasons'. The ding-dong battle between the *Miss Americas* and the *Miss Englands* ended there. During the previous five years, no less than seven records had been broken.

In 1933, Scott-Paine whose yard had built the first *Miss England* also tried to wrest the Harmsworth Trophy from Gar Wood in an aluminium speedboat called *Miss Britain III* – but without success. Indeed when the Trophy races were revived in 1949, Gar Wood's almost thirty-year-old tenure of the Trophy came to an end, merely because he was too old to compete.

# 14

## Diverse Legacy

The spirit of *Miss England II* was not to end there. In June 1932, Lady Doris Segrave wrote an article in the relatively new London journal 'Psychic News' entitled 'Sir Henry Segrave's Return'.

### "I know he is watching over me," says his widow.

Lady Segrave recounted how, in 1927, when her husband was making his attempt on the Land Speed Record at Daytona Beach, he received a message, given at a spiritualist seance in England. This was in the nature of a warning, said to have been given by a 'dead' speed king. In preventing a motoring accident that might have been fatal, this so aroused Segrave's curiosity that, on his return to England, the Major called on his friend Hannen Swaffer, whom he knew was interested in spiritualism. In Swaffer's well-lit flat, Segrave saw some psychic phenomena which made a deep impression on him. So much so that, in an article printed in the 'Sunday Express' a few days after he was killed, he was reported as saying, jokingly of course, "The only time I was ever frightened was when I saw the piano jump in Hannen Swaffer's flat."

Just after the fatal crash at Windermere, on Sunday 15th June, spontaneous phenomena occurred in Swaffer's flat which "suggested that Segrave was trying to prove his presence."

Swaffer wrote to Lady Segrave, describing in detail what had happened. She expressed appreciation. Then, a year later, she wrote to Swaffer having read one of his books on Spiritualism, and asked how she could inquire into it.

"One day Hannen Swaffer told me that he had received in the home circle of one of his friends, a message from my husband who said he was anxious to speak with me.

"I went to this home circle, where, for the first time since his death, I got in touch with my husband. I was so excited, and so was he, that I am afraid we spoiled this sitting, but there I received sufficient evidence to convince me of his survival after death.

"A few days later, a friend of Swaffer's, named Maurice Barbanell told me that he was going to a voice séance that night, and had arranged to take two friends with him. One of them was ill. Swaffer had asked him to get in touch with me, if ever he could manage to take me to a séance. Unfortunately I could not go that night. I had a very important engagement which could not be postponed."

According to Maurice Barbanell: "During that sitting the luminous trumpet moved towards me and a voice called my name. 'Who is that speaking?' I asked. The answer came, 'Segrave. Thank you for trying to bring my wife.' It was a perfect spirit message."

Lady Doris continued. "Later that evening he telephoned me again. He said my husband had been through with a message for me, which was certainly very characteristic, and that he also wanted to talk to me. Would I go to the next sitting?

"A fortnight afterwards I accompanied him to a house in Teddington. I was not introduced to the medium, or to any of the sitters. I learned afterwards that the medium was Mrs Estelle Roberts. With about fourteen others we went into a small room at the top of the house.

"The séance began with the singing of some hymns, and very soon afterwards a male voice spoke through one of the trumpets. They told me this was the voice of Red Cloud, the spirit guide who was in charge of the circle. The voice greeted some of his friends, and the conversations seemed very natural.

"The trumpet moved towards me and the voice said, 'You don't know me, do you?' – 'No,' I replied, 'I am a stranger here.' – 'Oh no you are not. Good evening Lady Segrave. I will soon bring your little man to you.'

"Another voice addressed me. 'D' it said. Only my husband had ever called me by that secret nickname. I became so tense that I could not speak. 'This is very difficult,' he went on, and the trumpet dropped to the ground. I was told this meant he could not 'hold the power'. Red Cloud immediately came through. 'I know how you feel,' he said 'and your husband is just as excited, but I will help you both.'

"I came away not knowing what to think. It seemed too good to be true.

"When I saw Mrs Roberts again, I asked her to give me a private trance sitting. She agreed, and it took place a few days later. It was full of evidence. It began with a message that proved conclusively that he was my husband. There followed so many details, names, incidents, the recalling of former conversations, that I knew beyond a shadow of doubt, I had found my husband again. One piece of evidence stands out in my memory. My husband again criticised my driving, reminding me of what he often used to say."

According to Barbanell, "Lady Segrave thereafter was a regular attendant. At séance after séance her husband gave her proof after proof. Soon, he was so perfect a communicator that he could bring the trumpet close to her ear and talk to her so that nobody else but she could hear."

Lady Segrave said, "Once, I asked permission to bring a

# "I KNOW HE IS WATCHING OVER ME," *says his Widow*

## By LADY SEGRAVE*

"I was a broken-hearted woman.

"Then I got proof of my husband's survival.

"Spiritualism removed all fear of death. It has brought me peace and comfort in my hour of trial.

"We used to be feted—cheering crowds—policemen clearing a way for our car, then . . . the world seemed to forget."

When my husband was making his attempt on the world's speed record at Daytona Beach, in 1927, he received a message, given at a séance in England,

A few days later, a friend of Swaffer's named Maurice Barbanell told me that he was going to a voice séance that night, and had arranged to take two friends with him. One of them was ill. Swaffer had asked him to get into touch with me, if ever he could manage to take me to a séance.

Unfortunately I could not go that night. I had a very important engagement, which could not be postponed. Later that evening he telephoned me again. He said my husband had been through with a message for me, which was certainly very characteristic, and that he also wanted to talk to me. Would I go to the next sitting ?

Press cutting on Segrave's "return". At each séance, Estelle Roberts was the clairvoyant medium through whom Segrave is said to have communicated from "beyond the grave".

friend, without mentioning his name. I wanted my husband to speak to Lord Cottenham, one of his oldest friends.

"The conversation between them at the next séance was an intimate and natural one. My husband told him of things that even I did not know. He called Lord Cottenham by his Christian name 'Mark', which no-one else there knew. It was obviously a re-union of old friends."

Barbanell verified this, saying that, "She got permission to bring two more strangers. Again, none of us knew who they were, but Segrave did! 'Rod' was his greeting to the young man. It was his brother Rodney. Segrave showed he knew who his companion was, for he called her by her name. She was his brother's wife.

"Lady Segrave told me how, after this sustained quest, she critically examined all her spirit messages, trying to explain them away. 'Always the evidence stood every test,' she said."

In July 1932 the Earl of Cottenham wrote a series of three articles for 'The Daily Express'. They were entitled 'My Introduction to Death', 'My Meeting with My Friend' and 'My Mediumship' in which he gave details of the development of his own powers.

People in the world of motoring and engineering science were astounded to read that Lord Cottenham had been convinced of the claims of Spiritualism. Cottenham was the sixth Earl. After leaving Charterhouse Public School, he studied engineering at Vickers Ltd. and London University. During the 1925 and 1926 Seasons at Brooklands Track, Cottenham, driving either an Austin Seven or a 'works' Alvis, raced against the ever successful Segrave in either a Darracq or a Talbot. Cottenham became Chairman of the Order of the Road, a motoring association he organised in order to promote safe driving.

At first, practically all the Earl knew of psychic matters was the result of staying with some Scottish friends, whom he regarded as fey. Then he accompanied Lady Segrave to Estelle Roberts' Teddington house to check things out. He attended several séances and 'Mark' and 'de Hane', as he and Segrave called each other, carried on, through the direct voice at Red Cloud's circles, very natural conversations. Soon after, Lord Cottenham discovered that he possessed psychic powers himself. Whilst sitting in his Buckinghamshire home, Maids Moreton Hall, he felt urged to write, and he found some outside force controlling his hand. Gradually, his automatic writing developed, and soon he decided to go public, "Otherwise I still read the reports of the classic motor races with deep interest. I drive my own touring car better than ever before, because de Hane Segrave is mentally with me ...

"My mother, my father, my brother, my friends Walter Seton and de Hane Segrave, every message they send me is couched in such wise, comforting and unselfish terms that it endorses – through their new point of view – the truth of a finer life, continuous with this one; a new section of life for which this earthly existence is but a school where the curriculum embraces every kind of good thought and action designed to make the school a better place.

"No psychic phenomenon I have witnessed, no experience I have had in or out of a séance room, no teaching that has come to me has done anything else but increase my belief in God."

To this day, there are some who say that spiritualist mediums are merely gifted with the power of telepathy to read the mind of their sitter and then invent the fact that the departed spirit of a loved one is communicating. To date, however, there has been no scientific proof put forward of telepathy.

\* \* \* \* \*

It is perhaps difficult nowadays to understand the impact that Segrave's death had upon the nation. There was neither Internet nor television and the deeds of those men and women of action who accomplished great things were brought to public attention by newspapers more concerned with reporting than digging up or inventing scandals about people in the public eye. Consequently, a very special niche was carved for many of these heroes in the hearts of the populace. So it was with Segrave.

Whilst researching this book, the author came into contact with several eye-witnesses to the Windermere accident. They had never forgotten the moment when the speedboat capsized. One of them, a teenage girl at the time, still kept an album of press cuttings forty years later.

In the autumn of 1930, the powers-that-be in motoring,

aviation and watersport, newspaper publishers and Segrave's friends – men like Lord Brabazon, Lord Howe, Lord Brecknock, Lord Sempill – and, of course, Lord Wakefield – got together and, with the consent of Lady Segrave, raised a trust fund to administer a trophy in his memory.

The task of creating a trophy, plaque and memorial worthy to bear the name Segrave was entrusted to a leading sculptor, Gilbert Bayes of St John's Wood, London. The original trustees of the Segrave Trophy were the Royal Automobile Club, the Royal Aero Club and the Marine Motoring Association. It was to be awarded to 'the British subject who, in the judgement of the Awarding Committee accomplishes the most outstanding demonstration of the possibilities of transport by land, air and water ... the simple idea behind this tribute to Sir Henry Segrave is to stimulate others also to uphold British prestige before the world by demonstrating how the display of courage, initiative and skill – the Spirit of Adventure itself – can assist progress in mechanical development ... '

During the past sixty-seven years, the Segrave Trophy has continued to be awarded to both men and women, ranging from long-distance aviators and aviatrixes, test-pilots, motor-racing champions and record-breaking drivers. Whilst its organisation has been taken care of by the Royal Automobile Club, sponsorship of the awards and award ceremony has been undertaken by such companies as Castrol and the Ford Motor Company.

The award was suspended during the Second World War, 1940-45; in other years where the trophy has not been awarded it has been because, in the opinion of the committee, there has been no achievement of sufficient merit to earn the award.

\* \* \* \* \*

On the afternoon of Saturday 19th October 1931, a memorial was unveiled to Vic Halliwell in the Parish churchyard of Portshead, his home town. The memorial was erected by Lord Wakefield "as a tribute to a brave man." It consisted of a Cenotaph-type headpiece in Dumbarton grey granite, with axed face for the lettering, which was in Roman style. It was surmounted by a bronze plaque, on which was modelled, in relief, *Miss England II* racing across the water, with a Schneider seaplane flying overhead. The work had been entrusted to the firm of J.N. Cox & Son of Cleveden, Michael Willcocks' home town.

## Winners of the Segrave Trophy

| | | | |
|---|---|---|---|
| 1930 | Sir Charles Kingsford Smith | 1977 | Barry Sheene |
| 1931 | Sqd. Ldr. Bert Hinkler | 1978 | Grp-Capt. John Cunningham |
| 1932 | Amy Johnson | 1979 | Mike Hailwood |
| 1933 | Sir Malcolm Campbell | 1980 | Lady Arran |
| 1934 | Ken Waller | 1982 | Rear-Admiral |
| 1935 | Capt G.E.T. Eyston | | Sandy Woodward |
| 1936 | Jean Batten | 1983 | Richard Noble |
| 1937 | Flying Officer A.E. Clouston | 1984 | Barry Sheene |
| 1938 | Major A.T. Goldie Gardner | 1985 | Wing-Commander Ken Wallis |
| 1939 | Sir Malcolm Campbell | 1986 | Richard Branson |
| 1946 | Geoffrey Raoul de Havilland | 1987 | Eve Jackson |
| 1947 | John Rhodes Cobb | 1988 | Martin Brundle |
| 1948 | John Douglas Derry | 1989 | Bob & Joe Ives |
| 1951 | Geoffrey Duke | 1990 | Louise Aitken Walker |
| 1953 | Sq. Ldr. Neville Duke | 1991 | Steve Webster |
| 1955 | Donald Campbell | 1992 | Frank Williams & N. Mansell |
| 1956 | Peter Twiss | 1993 | Eric Broadley |
| 1957 | Stirling Moss | 1994 | Carl Fogarty |
| 1958 | Donald Campbell | 1995 | Cohn McRae |
| 1960 | Tom Brooke-Smith | 1996 | Damon Hill |
| 1962 | A.W. Bedford | 1997 | Andy Green |
| 1964 | Donald Campbell | 1998 | Brian Milton |
| 1966 | Donald Campbell | 1999 | Jackie Stewart |
| 1968 | Wing-Commander Ken Wallis | 2002 | Steve Curtis |
| 1969 | Bruce McLaren | | |
| 1970 | Brian Trubshaw | | |
| 1973 | Jackie Stewart | | |
| 1974 | Major John Blashford Snell | | |
| 1975 | Roger Clark & Jim Porter | | |
| 1976 | Peter Collins | | |

Following a short and simple service in Portishead Parish church, the memorial was unveiled by Mr J.H. Inskip, Lord-Mayor Elect of Bristol. As two aeroplanes piloted by friends of Halliwell made a fly-past, dipping their wings in salute, Inskip pulled from the memorial the Union Jack which had fluttered, some sixteen months previously, from the stern of *Miss England II* at her official launching on Windermere. Among those present were Halliwell's widow and parents, and Michael Willcocks. In his address Inskip read the letter of tribute sent by His Majesty the King to Halliwell's father and describing the deceased engineer as 'your gallant son'.

In his book 'They Call it Courage – The Story of the Segrave Trophy', published in 1990, Phil Drackett wrote, "More than fifty years after Segrave's death on Windermere, a pensioner of the Castrol Company, living in Evesham, wrote to his former employers to the effect that in Portishead Churchyard, near Bristol, there was a grave in an unkempt state. The headstone indicated that it had been donated by Lord Wakefield, founder of the company. Under the circumstances, should not the company see that the grave was properly maintained? "Oh yes", he added, "the name on the headstone is Victor Halliwell ..."

For many years after the Windermere accident, on the 13th June, Harold Pattinson, who had been Clerk of the Course, went out in his motor-launch and placed a wreath on water at White Cross Bay, the site where Segrave had been fatally injured. Sir Henry's private sitting room at the nearby Old England Hotel, has ever since been known as the Segrave Room.

\* \* \* \* \* \*

Great Britain continued to pursue the highest speed across the water. Since 1922, Sir Malcolm Campbell had broken no less than twelve Land Speed Records in a series of increasingly powerful *Blue Bird* cars. In 1936 Campbell decided to have his first *Blue Bird* boat built by Saunders-Roe. He asked his Chief Mechanic, Leo Villa to go down to the bonded warehouse of LEP Transport, Chiswick where what was left of *Miss England II* was laid up. Villa collected boxes of shafts, props, air-starters, instruments and two large gearboxes.

Villa once recalled that at least one of these component parts was in the Rolls-Royce engined *Bluebird* single-step hydro-plane with which, in September 1937, Campbell succeeded in eclipsing Gar Wood's old record with a new average of 126.33mph across Italy's Lago Maggiore. The following year, *Bluebird* was taken to Lake Halwyl, Switzerland where she increased her speed to 130.9mph.

In 1939, with a second *Bluebird* hydroplane, still powered by a Rolls-Royce 'R' type but with a three-pointer hull configuration, Campbell further lifted his record to 141.17mph on Coniston Water, the lake adjacent to Windermere. Campbell superstitiously refused to run *Blue Bird* on Windermere, "... because Segrave was killed on that lake."

In 1947, when Campbell decided to convert his hydroplane to turbojet propulsion, he sold various parts of *Bluebird* (and formerly of *Miss England II*?) – gearbox, rudder, strut, shaft and propellers – to Maurice E. 'Bobby' Bothner of Johannesburg,

South Africa. Bothner's aim was to make an attempt on Campbell's 141mph record – but he found that the engine he had purchased was too powerful for his hull which became dangerously unstable at speeds approaching 150mph. He abandoned the project, bought a more conventional hydro in the USA and became one of the founding fathers in South African powerboat racing.

\* \* \* \* \*

In 1932, Michael Willcocks competed in his last motorboat race. A Mr J. King, owner of a Bristol tugboat company wanted an outboard raceboat. Willcocks introduced him to Fred Cooper, who designed him a boat to be powered by a Johnson 350cc B-Class outboard engine. The name of this plywood skiff was *Basileus* (Greek for king). The one and only time that *Basileus* was raced was at the 100-mile event on the River Bann, Belfast, Northern Ireland. Willcocks was at the helm: "I had the original wicker chair from *Miss England II* put in because my fractured spine was still painful." Today, *Basileus* has pride of place at the Motorboat Museum, near Basildon, Essex. During the decades that followed, Willcocks preserved that chair in the office of his family engineering company at Clevedon. In the late 1970s the author persuaded the ageing engineer to present this chair to the Windermere Steamboat Museum.

Also, thanks to Mr Charles Shephard, organiser of the International Power Boat Grand Prix in the Bristol Docks, the 'Segrave Salver' was donated by Michael Willcocks, who presented it on the first occasion in memory of his skipper.

\* \* \* \* \*

In 1938, Gabriele d'Annunzio died from a cerebral haemorrhage, at his worktable in the Vittoriale. In June 1951, thirteen years later, the Ninth Regatta for the Oltranza Cup was held on Lake Garda. Among those invited to take part were Sir Malcolm Campbell's son, Donald, in the Rolls-Royce-engined *Bluebird* prop-rider, and a Windermere solicitor by the name of Norman Buckley in his Jaguar XK120-engined hydroplane *Miss Windermere II*. Campbell won the Oltranza Cup for the two fastest laps at 156 km/h and the roar of a Rolls-Royce aero-engine echoed off the walls of d'Annunzio's stone mausoleum in the

gardens of the Vittoriale. Norman Buckley became the first Englishman to win a post-war powerboat race outside England.

Buckley was later to recall a strange irony about that contest:
"Present that day on Garda were myself, Donald Campbell, the
two Italian pilots Ezio Selva and Mario Verga. John Cobb,
current holder of the World Land Speed Record and preparing
for an attack on the Water Speed Record, had come as an interested spectator.

"In 1952 Cobb was killed when his speedboat disintegrated
at 240mph on Loch Ness. In 1954, Verga was killed with his
Alfa-Romeo-engined speedboat took off at near record speed.
Selva took one of the Alfa-Romeo engines out of Verga's
wrecked hydroplane saying that one engine could not kill two
men. But then in 1958, Selva was killed in that same boat at the
Orange Bowl Regatta race in Miami, Florida. Donald Campbell
was killed on Coniston Water in 1967 when his jet-engined
*Bluebird K7* failed to completely loop the loop at almost
300mph. Now I am the only one alive."

Ironically, Norman Buckley died in 1975 during an operation for a double hernia. It is a saga that would surely have
appealed to d'Annunzio.

*Miss England II*'s engine-less and badly damaged hull
remained in the Chiswick warehouse of LEP Transport.
Although rumours circulated for a long time that she was
languishing in the barn of a Yorkshire farm, the truth was that
she was eventually demolished by a grouping of Nazi fire-bombs sometime in 1940. For wartime security reasons, it was not possible to name either people or companies but a cutting from page 3 of the 'Brentford and Chiswick

**Incendiaries Again.**

Incendiary bombs, some half a dozen in number, were dropped in a western district on another night, but only one of them suc-ceeded in causing anything like a fire, and that was put out in about a quarter of an hour. One of the missiles dropped through a craft owned by a man whose name was famous in the motor boat racing world some few years ago. Again the fire-fighting ser-vices proved their efficiency for, although calls were many, they were on the spot quickly, and thus were able to limit the damage done to a very small degree; that was one of the comparatively quiet nights.

*Miss England II* was housed at LEP, Chiswick. The press article from the Brentford and Chiswick Times, dated 4th October 1940, describes her destruction *(London Borough of Hounslow)*

Times' for 4th October 1940 entitled 'Incendiaries Again' seems to detail the ultimate destruction of a boat which, just one decade before, had been a legend of tragic success.

## Is there anything left of *Miss England II*?

Visitors to d'Annunzio's Vittoriale degli Italiani, open to the General Public since 1975, and preserved exactly as it was at the poet's death in 1938, can still be given a guided visit to the Priory and enter the Relics Room, where from a distance they can see Segrave's twisted steering wheel, surrounded by Madonnas and Buddhas. Her deck hatch is still proudly displayed on the wall of the Windermere Motor Boat Racing Clubhouse.

## Models of *Miss England II*

Whilst one-off scale models were made of this speedboat, it was not until 1948 that the name 'Miss England' was used on a toy. This was a 13½-inch long silver and red "Super Toy Speed Boat" manufactured for only one year by Victoria Industries (Surrey) Ltd. It was steam-driven, fired by a methylated spirit burner and in no way resembled the three white namesakes which had made the headlines almost twenty years before. Then, from the early 1990s, model-maker Fred Harris of Southport, having carefully researched plans of *Miss England II*, has been making 1/43rd scale models in kit or ready-built forms. In addition, in the late 1990s, Fred Harris built three metre-long (1/12th scale) models of this legend. One of them stands alongside this writer's computer today, one went to the USA, and the third was sold at Christie's for £2,225.

To date, no-one has built a full-scale replica of what many have described as the most beautiful British speedboat of the 1930s.

# Appendix

## Bibliography

*Il Vittoriale*, Annamaria Andreoli (Electa, Milano, 1993)

*The Schneider Trophy Races*, Ralph Barker (Chatto and Windus, 1971)

*Speed Boat Kings*, J. Lee Barrett (Arnold-Powers Inc., 1939)

*Kaye Don – the Man*, James Wentworth Day (Hutchinson, 1934)

*Guinness Book of Motorboating Facts & Feats*, Kevin Desmond (Guinness Superlatives Ltd., 1978)

*Power Boat Speed*, Kevin Desmond (Conway Maritime Press,1987)

*They Call it Courage*, Phil Drackett (Robert Hale, 1990)

*Pui oltre, Gabriele d'Annunzio et la motonautica*, Vittorio Pirlo (Edizione e cura dell'Associazione Culturale l'Oleandro, 1994)

*Sir Henry Segrave*, Cyril Posthumus (Batsford, 1961)

*Fast Boats and Flying Boats*, Adrian Rance (Ensign, 1989)

*The World Water Speed Record*, Leo Villa & Kevin Desmond (Batsford, 1976)

### Acknowledgements:

Interviews with M.J. Willcocks, R.E. Garner and other members of the *Miss England II* team.

For additional research and illustrations: Archivi Fondazione 'Il Vittoriale degli Italiani'; The Motorboat Museum, Basildon; National Motor Museum, Beaulieu.

## *Also from Sigma Leisure:*

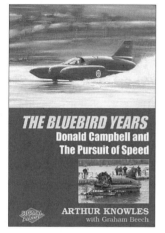

### THE BLUEBIRD YEARS:
### Donald Campbell and the Pursuit of Speed
*Arthur Knowles, with Graham Beech*
This best-seller is a gripping description of Donald Campbell's attempts to propel his *Bluebird* jet-boat faster than 300mph. It contains Arthur Knowles's 1967 account of Campbell's preparations and his final tragic attempt, plus new material and photographs by co-author Graham Beech on the recovery of the wreck and the funeral of Donald Campbell in 2001. The challenges that faced the designers of *Bluebird* are described, together with an analysis of the causes of the crash by Ken Norris, co-designer of *Bluebird*. Listings of water-speed records, the technology required for timing record attempts and updates on the latest challengers are all included. The human story is also featured, with background on the Campbell family and the continuing *Bluebird* heritage.   *£9.95*

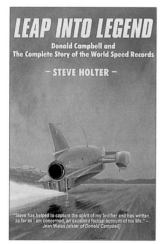

### LEAP INTO LEGEND: Donald Campbell and the complete story of The World Speed Records
*Steve Holter*
Here are the life stories of the most famous British record breakers: Donald Campbell and his father, Sir Malcolm. It is also a story of the triumphs of British engineering between the two world wars, when huge aeroengines were being developed for the war effort, and ultimately used in peacetime to drive record-breaking cars and boats. While the Campbells take pride of place, the successes and failures of many others are also chronicled – the dates, times and places plus the official and unofficial speed records on land, water and even in space.
Includes details of the tragic death of Donald Campbell in 1967, and reliable information on the many *Bluebird* cars, boats and planes built and destroyed during the 20th century.   *£10.95*

**All of our books are available through booksellers. In case of difficulty, or for a free catalogue, please contact: SIGMA LEISURE, 5 ALTON ROAD, WILMSLOW, CHESHIRE SK9 5DY**
Phone: 01625-531035
E-mail: info@sigmapress.co.uk
Web site: http//www.sigmapress.co.uk

# Limited Edition Prints of Paintings by Arthur Benjamins

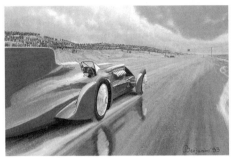

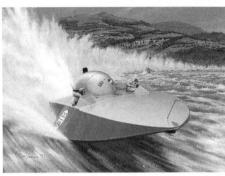

**"One Hell of a Job"**: Malcolm Campbell in the 1933 *Blue Bird* on Daytona Beach. Print size 19" x 25"

**"And to Hell with You Too"**: Donald Campbell at the helm of *Blue Bird K4* during the 1950 Oltranza Cup Race. Print size 19" x 23"

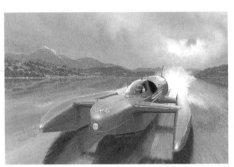

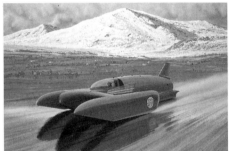

**"Full Power"**: Donald Campbell with *Bluebird K7* on Coniston Water during 1966. Print size 19" x 25"

**"The Christmas Run"**: *Bluebird K7* passing the Old Man of Coniston. Print size 18" x 25"

| | | |
|---|---|---|
| **One Hell of A Job**, unsigned | £25 |
| Signed and numbered by the artist | £45 |
| | |
| **And to Hell with you Too**, unsigned | £25 |
| Signed and numbered by the artist | £45 |
| | |
| **Full Power**, unsigned | £25 |
| Signed and numbered by the artist | £45 |
| Signed and numbered by the artist, and countersigned by Mr Ken Norris | £85 |
| Signed & numbered by the artist, and countersigned by both Mr Ken Norris & Mrs Jean Wales | £125 |
| | |
| **The Christmas Run**, unsigned | £25 |
| Signed and numbered by the artist | £45 |
| Signed and numbered by the artist, and countersigned by Mr Ken Norris | £85 |

*Further information on these and other prints can be obtained from:*
Blue Bird Publications, 162 Swievelands Road, Biggin Hill, Kent TN16 3QX, UK.
Tel: 01959 574414; Fax: 01959 571077; e-mail: bbirdpubl@aol.com

Orders, with cheques payable to "Blue Bird Publications" should be sent to the above address. Post & packing for each order: UK £5.50. Europe £8. Worldwide £15.